MY JOURNEY WITH

JOSIE

A Sister's Memoir of a Family's Struggle with Terminal Cancer

Salvina Grice

To Elizabeth
May our journey
guide you to live
your life with
hope and gratitude
Salvina Grice
July 2014.

Produced by:

FriesenPress
Suite 300 – 852 Fort Street
Victoria, BC, Canada V8W 1H8

www.friesenpress.com

Distributed to the trade by The Ingram Book Company

Table of Contents

This book was written
in loving memory of my sister Josie
and is dedicated to her three children
Anthony, Paul and Andrea.

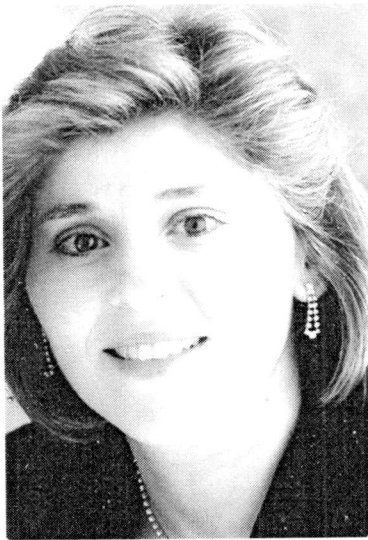

A Mother's love is never forgotten
July 18th 1955-May 14th 1995

Acknowledgements

THIS IS usually the part of a book that I quickly skip over to get to the good stuff. As embarrassed as I am to admit this, it is true. Now that I have endured the process of pouring my thoughts, feelings and life experiences onto paper, I realize the true value of this section. The writing of My Journey with Josie was made possible by so many people here, there and everywhere. But the message was sent to me on a summer night when good friends old and new, Rocco, Ken, Brian and Gratz, came together at our place for dinner and drinks. It was a gorgeous summer night and as the discussions evolved, we realized that we were not alone. There was magic all around us and a deep sense of comfort in knowing that our loved ones were not so far away. That night set me on a new path in my life that would take me on this spiritual journey and I will be forever grateful.

This book would have never been completed if it were not for my husband Chris, whose support and encouragement have been endless. I appreciate you protecting my time, screening my calls, picking up the slack and for always ensuring that I had a hot cup of tea on my side table. For this and so much more, I will always love you.

Speaking of picking up the slack, I want to acknowledge my two beautiful children who have literally kept me going in my life during times when I felt I couldn't. I thank you both for being patient and supportive. I know that during this process, I missed quite a few of your hockey games Mitch. Although you enjoyed teasing me and making me feel guilty for that, you ought to know that whether I am near or far, I am always cheering for you. I love you and respect the commitment that you bring to everything that you do. I am proud to call you my son.

Nicole, you are my beautiful daughter with all your special gifts. I know that our chick nights have been few and far between lately, but your understanding and encouragement has never wavered. I know that you have believed in me and my ability to write this book from the start. Count me in to do the same when you are writing your first novel. Nicole, I appreciate your view of the world and for teaching me so much about being a mother. I love you and I thank you.

Thank you to my other sister, Tina who gave me the space but somehow always knew when I needed her. I am so blessed to have you in my life and grateful that we have come so far.

Many thanks to my extended family for their continued enthusiasm and support. A special mention to Mary Anne for helping with the final touches.

I also want to thank you Cecilia for your commitment and passion during the writing of My Journey with Josie. You were always there for me and encouraged me to find my truth. I look forward to many more years of friendship.

Thank you to Kelly for your support and ongoing encouragement. You are one of the most thoughtful people that I have ever known. Where would we all be without friends?

Thanks Joanne for meeting with me and sharing some of your fondest memories of Josie. I am so glad that Josie's dearest friends, Marnie and Franca were also able to meet. It was so great to get together and reminisce about Josie and how much she meant to us. It almost felt like she was with us. I guess we carry around a little piece of Josie wherever we go. That is true friendship.

My acknowledgements would not be complete without thanking my beautiful black and white tuxedo cat, Quinney. There were many times in writing this book that I wept and sobbed and laughed and cried and he lay beside me giving me comfort and support and never asking, "Mom whats for dinner? You are my little cat-man.

Of course my greatest inspiration for this book was my love and commitment to Josie's children, Anthony, Paul and Andrea. Your mother was the definition of love and grace. She would want you to know that you always came first in her life and that you deserve the best that life has to offer. In a short amount of time, your mother gave all three of you a lifetime of love and learning that is evident in the people that you have all come to be. Thank you for being in my life and sharing the light of your mother that shines through each of you every day.

I would like to thank and acknowledge my family in spirit for their protection and their guidance. Thank you all for showing me in your subtle and not so subtle ways, that I am not alone and that I have not been abandoned or forgotten. I am loved.

Finally, to Josie I thank you for always loving me and for giving me the strength, the courage, and often times the words to have made My Journey with Josie possible.

Introduction

To you my reader, my sincere gratitude for opening these pages and being a part of My Journey with Josie. Writing this book has been a labor of love and a very personal journey. I feel that I have let go and freed myself of the pain that has held me back for so long. Initially, I decided to write this book because through Spirit, Josie asked me to tell her story. I thought it would be a privilege for me to write about her and leave a legacy for her children. I felt so blessed that I was able to do this for her and for them. However, as I became more involved in our story, I realized that there was so much more.

Since Josie's passing, I have come to know that I must let her go. In some ways I feel that I have, just by living my life without her. But truthfully, I really have not known how to let her go. Her loss has been deep rooted in me for years, in a place that I haven't been able to reach but I keep trying to fill. The pain of losing Josie has not only kept me overweight, but has kept me feeling alone and in constant fear.

I have always feared change because the events that have altered my life the most have been when I lost those that I love. I have learned so much about myself, so it has become my intention to help others do the same. By reading about my personal challenges, I hope that you all can laugh, cry, and come away with your own sense of personal freedom. I know that for all of these years I have been stuck, but I am now ready to release myself , and in doing so, I will allow Josie's spirit the freedom to spread her own wings and fly.

MY JOURNEY WITH
JOSIE

**A Sister's Memoir of a Family's
Struggle with Terminal Cancer**

Chapter 1

A New Beginning

IS MY worst nightmare about to repeat itself like the old Star Trek dreams I used to have every night when I was a kid? Trapped on that strange looking airplane and not being able to get off, and thinking that I would never be able to see my family and my friends again. I am on the phone with the nurse and can't believe what I am hearing. I need to pull myself together and catch my breath for a moment. I ask the nurse to repeat herself. It sounds like she is telling me something about a cyst on my right ovary and that I have lots of fibroid, but she can't possibly be talking about me. Ok just breathe. I look for the closest seat possible. It is all that I can do to keep myself from falling over.

I hear the voice say, "Mrs. Grice, the ultrasound also shows that the lining of your uterus is very thick". But I can't respond. I don't understand.

"How the hell does the lining of your uterus get thick?" I ask. I already know that nothing good can come of this conversation.

"Would that explain why I have been bleeding for the past three weeks?" I ask. I thought I was making up for the period that I missed the previous month. You know, heaven forbid

1

that I get away with something without any consequences.

"It's possible" she answers

I was hoping that this missed period meant the end of it forever. Obviously I am getting way ahead of myself. What makes me so special? I too have to endure the whole menopausal ordeal like the rest. Perhaps I am over reacting, and anyways, I have to go back to work. I try to shut it out of my mind but I can't stop thinking of my mom, who over thirty years ago went in for a routine hernia operation and came out with cancer of the uterus. Or was it her ovaries? I really don't know which to this day. Does it really matter? I guess it does to me right now. Have I followed in her path?

"We need to book you in to see a gynecologist" The nurse says in her sweetest voice possible. "Do you have a preference?" I try to speak but the words get caught in my throat. I try to compose myself. "Mrs. Grice, do you have a particular preference or someone in mind?"

"I don't know" I respond at last "I'll get back to you. Thank you". Of course I am very polite. Maybe I even sound too professional. Once I hang up the phone my head won't stop spinning. How can this be happening to me? I have always thought of myself as someone who could handle just about everything and in many ways, I have been through my fair share. Life has not always been kind, and here I am once again, feeling very afraid and unsure about what lay ahead of me.

Summer has just ended. It has been the most productive summer that I have ever had. I finally followed through on making some of the hard decisions in my life. I have gotten myself into an exercise program and I am actually swimming in my pool more than my kids. I even have a personal trainer. I know that sounds so glamorous, but really she is my massage therapist. Oh, that sounds kind of ippity too but really Theresa is great. She is a military woman who was deployed overseas. She has a strong build, takes care of her body and keeps herself in good shape. She can be real tough but her round face, blue eyes and warm smile tell a different story. She comes to my house three times a week to teach me to do exercises in the pool at no charge. She is a very kind and generous person. You know there are some really good people in this world, and she is one of them. I even stopped smoking. I had been smoking for nineteen years and I finally quit, only finding out that I'm dying anyways?

I decide to pick myself up as I always do and do what I do best; talk. Only I talk myself into the worst case scenario possible. I imagine myself talking to my doctor, my husband and children, family and friends about this cancer that will eventually take complete control of me. After all, isn't that what cancer does? Prey on the strong and the innocent? It leaves behind a path of destruction resulting in fear, blame, pain and unquenchable anger. Anger, that leads to loneliness and sadness that is deep-rooted, in the depths of your soul. The kind that lingers, hanging over you like a cloud on a gloomy day reminding you of what you once held so dear. This is the scenario that I am all too familiar with.

My thoughts are almost too much to bear. I can't help but hold my head in my hands and cry, wondering, not knowing, how everyone especially my husband and my children, will ever survive without me. Suddenly, in the midst of all the chaos I have created in my head, emerges this feeling that in the end, I am going to be okay. I have to stay positive. I have to be strong for my family. After all, I have been feeling well and my appetite is fine too. I've never had any problems there. I haven't really lost any weight, only inches, but that's because of all the exercising I've been doing. Things are going to be just fine won't they?

I feel that I am a loving wife, a caring mother, and a loyal friend. I would do anything for anyone. I have worked hard, dedicating my life to helping children and families in need. My work hasn't always been easy, but it has its personal rewards too.

I pull into my parking space at work and I know that I have to collect myself; I check my complexion in the mirror. I look tired and a little pale. I take a deep breath of fresh air as I exit the car, collect my bag, and slam the car door. Today is going to be a long day but I know I can make it through. I smile at myself in the reflection of the car window. Willing myself to be happy and stay positive. I make sure to have an extra big smile on my face for good measure.

I know I can do this but my mind wanders back to the negative. I have seen this happen too often in my life within my own family. I want to get back on that scary Star Trek plane and zoom my way to some other galaxy where I don't have to deal with any of this. So much for the person that has always faced life's challenges head on. I will admit that I want to escape what I fear is ahead of me. But I know that I need to be brave and go through this, whatever this is, in the same way that I preach to others. Be positive and stop thinking the worst. And thinking is what I do.

Chapter 2

Patience Is A Virtue

I CALL MY family doctor's office back with the name of a gynecologist who came highly recommended by my friend Kelly.

"Yes hello" I hear myself say when the receptionist finally answers the phone. "This is Mrs. Grice calling back. I was asked to call back with the name of a gynecologist; may I speak with the nurse please?" I ask.

"Certainly, please hold". I wait on the phone for several minutes before a woman with an assertive tone answers the phone. I tell her that I would like to see a gynecologist by the name of Dr. Patel and she assures me that she will get to work on it right away.

"Thank you Mrs. Grice. I will call their office and make an appointment for you and fax over a copy of your ultra sound results. You will likely have to have a biopsy taken by the gynecologist."

"Biopsy?" I reply with an alarming tone in .my voice.

"Yes, we need to take a biopsy as a precaution". A precaution for what, cancer I think to myself? Just the thought of that word brings about a hollow feeling in the pit of my stomach.

I take a deep breath and calmly say, "Did I mention that I am still bleeding?"

She tells me that the prolonged bleeding is very common and that most women continue to bleed for this long. What reassurance this offers I am not sure. She also suggests that I check on the internet to determine what iron enriched foods I should eat

"Oh and take some iron supplements. Any over the counter will do" she adds. I am not impressed. I suppose the fact that I am feeling weaker everyday and more and more fatigued isn't enough. I am also feeling a shortness of breath that I have never experienced before. Not even when I was in my twenties and smoking a pack of cigarettes a day. The nurse assures me this is normal and the blood tests I had taken a week ago did not show any iron deficiencies.

She does not even recommend that I come in to see the doctor. I am growing more pissed off with each passing minute of this conversation. I'm bleeding to death can't she see that? How can she not care?

I have to remind myself that it's not her fault, yet somehow I blame her anyways. I end the conversation abruptly and hang up. I put the phone down on the table and lay my face down on the cold granite and sigh. No one is really taking me seriously so I begin to doubt myself again. Perhaps I am making too much of this, but honestly I feel like I am dying a slow death.

As the days pass and I wait for my appointment with the gynecologist, I have moments when I feel calm. It is either that quiet voice reassuring me that all will be fine, or that my iron levels are so low I don't have the energy to even worry about it. At any rate, I am feeling hopeful, less alert, but hopeful. That's a good start in my mind.

Another week has passed and I have not heard from the gynecologist's office. I mention this to my sister Tina, who has been checking in on me with her daily phone calls.

"What do you mean you haven't gotten a call back yet? It's been a week" you can hear the frustration rising in her voice. "Well, if I were you I'd call the office and see what is taking so long. It's not like it's hard to set an appointment and call you back".

"I know" I reply, trying to sound equally annoyed, but not being able to muster the strength to really care anymore. "You're right. I'll call as soon as we're finished our conversation". This seems to satisfy her, and I smile as I think of how fortunate I am to have a sister as thoughtful and caring as she is.

I hang up the phone and I contact the gynecologist's office to find out why it is taking so long to book my appointment. Apparently, the fax was sent by my family doctor to the gynecologist and an appointment was set for four weeks from now.

" Four weeks, are you kidding me?" I cry. "Perhaps there are some things you may not be aware of. First of all, I have been bleeding for over a month. It is heavy and it is steady. Secondly, my mother was diagnosed with ovarian or uterine cancer at the age of fifty-eight. I am now forty eight. As for the rest of it, I can assure you that I have an extensive family history of cancer. What is wrong with you people`` I shout. By this point my composure goes out the window and I start hyperventilating. "My father and my..."

"Mrs. Grice, we had no idea that you had such a history" The nurse cuts in.

"I cannot wait the four weeks" I sob. Fortunately she is very sympathetic to my situation and advises me that this important information was not faxed over to their office. Finally, she suggests that I contact my family doctor's office and request that the information be sent. How on earth could this information be missed? I feel totally exasperated and frustrated with this process. I am slowly losing faith in our health care system as now I need to contact my family doctor's office once again.

I am totally not willing to have this conversation but I know that I have to. I dial the number and wait to be connected to the nurse who finally answers the phone. I ask her to explain why my family history was not faxed over to the gynecologist. Of course she denies this and assures me that all of my family medical history, including my test results were definitely faxed over. Obviously someone is not telling the truth and I know that it is her. In an effort to rectify the situation, she quickly agrees to resend all of my information. I decide to never return to that family doctor's office again.

I hang up the phone and feel the whole room spinning and my breath is becoming shallow. I am beginning to really worry about how this is all going to end. I sit down in my comfy brown leather recliner and pull my feet up on the foot rest. I grab my favorite blanket as I always do and close my eyes. Why don't they understand how serious this is?

Chris is out of town for work and I am working too. But driving around is getting risky. I feel so light headed. The other night I was driving home from the parent- teacher barbeque at Nikki's school and I almost ran a child over. I decided then and there that driving a car was not an option for me at this time.

My sister Tina phones me and when I tell her how weak I feel, she begs me to go to the emergency. Unfortunately, she works across the city and can't take me. This is definitely a time when you need a trusted friend. So I call my co-worker, Kelly who agrees I should go and God bless her, offers to take me.

Kelly and I arrive at the hospital and wait for my name to be called. After a surprisingly short time, I am called in by a handsome male nurse and am ushered into an examination room for blood tests. As it turns out, Kelly went to high school with him. What a small world it is. Despite being in an emergency ward, I find the experience to be rather pleasant; the staff seems to be very caring and friendly. We chat as we wait for my blood results. When the doctor arrives he too is very friendly and approachable. He shares the results of my blood test and tells me that my iron levels are dangerously low and gives me medication to stop the bleeding at least until I see the gynecologist.

My appointment with him is a week from now and I can't wait to get this over with. That's the good news. The bad news is that after a week, the pills are doing nothing for me and my flow is still going strong. What the heck is going on?

I decide that a warm shower is definitely what I need to relax and wash away my worries. I slip out of my robe, allowing it to fall into a heap on the floor. I step into the tub and pull the curtain closed. I feel my muscles relax instantly and my mind begins to wander. I ask myself why women have to go through so much pain and humiliation in their lifetime. It starts so early in our lives and many of us aren't even teenagers when we are first introduced to our new "friend".

What's all the buzz about anyways, babies? Many of us know what happens during childbirth. More pain and humiliation and more sacrifices. I realize that I sound terribly negative. There is no greater joy than bringing a child into this world and being that child's mother, I know this first hand. But the sleepless nights, the struggle to fit back into your clothes, and of course, the one year wait until you feel like yourself again. All of this only to get menopause when it all shuts down and a whole new set of problems begin? Have I made my point? I am just tired, scared and pissed!

Chapter 3

Getting Through It

CHRIS TOOK the day off work to bring me to the appointment and be there for moral support. I really do appreciate the sentiment, and besides we both know that I am in no condition to be driving.

"Mrs. Grice?" I hear a voice calling my name. It's the nurse. She seems friendly and escorts me and Chris into one of the private examination rooms. As we are walking down the hallway Chris squeezes my hand; he knows that I am feeling nervous. I can sense that he is too and I squeeze back. Our eyes meet as we enter the room and Chris helps me to find my seat. After answering a few questions, the nurse tells me that the doctor will be in shortly and leaves the room.

"Babe it's all going to be fine" Chris assures me. His droopy brown eyes look so tired. He has been working so much lately and feeling little satisfaction. His shaggy salt and pepper hair frame his handsome face well. He and I have been through so much together.

Before I even have a chance to answer, Dr. Patel walks into the room and I feel my body tighten. I am told that Dr. Patel is a wonderful doctor. He appears to be much younger than me, but then again it seems like a lot of people are younger than me these days. Dr. Patel is from India but he was clearly born here. His dark wavy hair and light brown skin compliment his good looks and I would guess that he is in his mid to late thirties.

"Good morning Mrs. Grice. I am Dr. Patel. How are you feeling?" he asks. His voice is one of the kindest that I have heard in a long time. I feel a certain calm when I am talking with him.

"Well I have seen better days" I say with a chuckle. "I have been taking the medication that was given to me, but it has not stopped the bleeding as it was supposed to". I go on to explain how weak I have been feeling and how difficult it is becoming to function on a daily basis. "The bleeding is still so heavy and I don't know what else to do" I add sounding desperate for a solution.

Dr. Patel goes on to discuss my ultrasound results and explains that his main concern is the thickening of the endometrial lining of my uterus, as that is where all the bleeding is coming from. He suggests that a biopsy be taken to determine the cause.

I have had a lot of gynecologists in my lifetime to deal with my endometriosis as well as various other things. However, no one has been as compassionate or as kind. He is very gentle and tries to make me feel as comfy as possible. In spite of his efforts I am still terrified and embarrassed when I think about laying there with my legs wide open.

I knew before arriving for this appointment that I would have a biopsy, but here I am and it's happening for real. For the doctor to want to take a biopsy, that must mean he is just as worried as I am.

"Oh, are you thinking that it is cancerous?" I ask with fear in my voice.

"Well no but the biopsy will rule out the possibility of cancer. There is no doubt that you have been losing a lot of blood and your iron is very low, but we must not jump to conclusions at this point Mrs. Grice". In a calming and reassuring tone, he asks me to remove my clothing from the waist down and get comfortable on the table until he returns. I agree and Dr. Patel leaves the room.

Chris helps me out of my clothes and into the dressing gown that is provided. We wait for Dr. Patel to return. I sense Chris getting anxious and we look into each other's eyes. Chris asks me if he could wait outside in the waiting room during the procedure. I need to think about this for a moment and hesitate, but there really is no time because I hear Dr. Patel talking to his nurse outside the door.

"Go ahead" I reply hastily "I'll see you when I'm done".

"Are you sure? I'll stay if you prefer it's just" I cut him off mid sentence.

"No it's fine, just go".

Is this another scenario where I am feeling abandoned and unsupported? Or is Chris just being a woosie and is terrified at the sight of blood. I am thinking that he does not want to embarrass himself in front of me or the good doctor.

I am still bleeding as I gingerly lower myself onto the examination table. There are splatters of blood everywhere and I look up at Dr. Patel utterly helpless as he enters the room. There is nothing I can do about it, but the whole experience is just so humiliating. Dr. Patel looks back at me with compassion as if to say "its okay, things are going to be fine". I feel so vulnerable but at least his look helps to quell some of the fear that I feel rising up inside of me.

This is definitely one of those times that I need to be brave. I clench my fists and hold my breath as I lay there thinking about the fact that I have bled month after month for every period since I was twelve, and now I am going to go out bleeding right till the end. I want it to be over before he even starts but I know that I am in good hands.

In the midst of my apprehension, I suddenly hear this little voice telling me, "You will get through this". Before I realize what I have just heard, I am cranked open and my insides are pricked and pinched with what seems like a very sharp object.

I lay there with tears rolling down my face but I am relieved that it is over and I did get through it just like the voice said I would.

After pulling myself together, Dr. Patel asks me to see the nurse who books his surgeries.

"Surgery?" I ask, surprised.

"Yes Mrs. Grice. I think that it is necessary and I recommend that you have a full hysterectomy" He responds confidently.

I'm not sure what to say, wondering if a hysterectomy will really stop all the bleeding, so I ask, "Will my bleeding stop as a result of this surgery?"

"Yes, I am certain that a full hysterectomy will fix the problem. Mrs. Grice the reason we should opt for the full hysterectomy is because it would be beneficial to remove your ovaries as well, given your family history".

Chris is waiting for me in the waiting room and jumps up from his seat when he sees me. I look up at him and he has this look on his face, a bit sheepish at first. I can tell that he may have regretted his decision to not be there to hold my hand. He looks so scared. I'm sure he is thinking the worst of what could happen to me and what his life would be like without me. I know that I have these thoughts too. I suppose I could really build up the procedure to have been one of the worst and loneliest times of my life, when I needed him and he let me down. But I decide not to even though the procedure was no picnic. I've been through so much heartache in my life already and this just seems like one more thing. I tell Chris that the doctor is recommending a full hysterectomy.

"He needs to remove my uterus to stop the bleeding and given my family history, the ovaries need to come out too."

Chris has really been going through a lot of his own challenges these days and you can see the wearing down on his face. He seems shocked that surgery is necessary and asks "Are you okay?"

"Yes I will be" I assure him even though I really don't know for sure. He puts his arms around me and I feel the warmth of his body giving me strength. He takes my hand and we walk together to meet the nurse.

The nurse who books the surgeries is the nicest person. She is very kind and willing to go the extra mile to find a spot for me.

"Dr. Patel has no surgery space open for a while" she states.

"How much longer do I have to wait" I ask in anticipation of the shortest amount of time possible.

"I need to borrow some surgery time from one of the other gynecologists. Dr. Patel told me to get you in as soon as possible because your situation is urgent".

Finally someone is taking me seriously. This Dr. Patel is a saint and I must remember to thank Kelly for the recommendation.

"I will call you back to let you know when I have a time available".

"That's great, thank you so much" I reply. It seems like surgery is the only way to stop this bleeding. That will be a relief.

On the drive home in the car, I think of all that has happened this morning and I feel good that I am finally getting closer to getting through this just like that little voice had whispered in my ear earlier today.

The bad news is that my problem is urgent and to me that means it is really serious. Oh I'm so tired of all this and it has only just begun. I need a nap when we get home. But how can I even think of sleeping, not knowing what will happen to me and my children? What about Chris? How will he manage? My siblings, my nieces and nephews, I mean something to all these people don't I? I feel myself dozing in the car, my eye lids getting heavy in spite of my effort to stay awake.

It is a dreary day but that suits me and my mood just fine. We finally make it home and I make myself comfortable on the recliner. In the meantime, I have to wait for this nice woman whose name I can't even remember to call me as soon as she finds a three hour time slot as that is how long the surgery will likely take. Until then all I can do is worry. My breast reduction surgery was three hours long and *that* was considered major surgery. I guess this is too.

Chapter 4

The Time Is Now

I AM LOSING track of time. Sleeping in a comatose state is something I am getting used to. You know that sleep state when your eyes are open and you can hear what is going on around you, but you can't lift a finger because you are too weak and your body feels so heavy? This feeling is becoming my reality. My condition is deceiving however, even Dr. Patel thought I looked great when he saw me. He said that he would have never guessed that my iron levels had dropped as low as they had by looking at me.

I have always had the rosiest cheeks and for my whole life I have hated that. This is one time I am grateful for having a touch of rosacea. But it hasn't lasted long; my iron deficiency is really starting to show. I can see this dull yellowness on my face and it's kind of freaking me out.

Yesterday the nurse called back, and I am booked for a full hysterectomy a week from today. I have to do the usual pre-op — great more blood tests. Is there going to be any left?

It has been almost a month that I have not been at work. I made all the necessary calls to my manager as well as to human resources. I was told that I need to provide a note, but I am not worried about any of that. You know when you are really sick it is all that you think about day and night and *that* is all that becomes important.

Even with the kids I have not signed agendas, read the millions of notes that have come home, or even checked to see if homework was being done. I am usually right on top of that. It is like I have surrendered all my responsibilities. I know the kids are concerned. They haven't admitted this to me but I know. I have always done so much for them and now it's all come to a halt.

I explained as much as I could without too much detail because my son gets very woozie like his dad -- No dreams of him becoming a doctor. And my daughter has only been getting her "friend" for a year and so far is following my path. So I don't want to totally freak her out. I want to protect my children by not telling them the whole truth. But really, what is the truth? Even I am uncertain. I assured them that I am going to be just fine as any good mother would.

I tell them that I will only be in the hospital for a night, and then I hope to be up and about after that in no time. I do not know any of this to be true but I tell them anyway. Things are happening so quickly and I realize that I don't even know the results of my biopsy. I have finished my prescription and I am still bleeding.

Chris is working all day and then coming home and taking care of me and the kids. Even though that is what I have always done, somehow women make it look so much easier. Surprisingly I have the meals prepared. I do them in stages a little bit at a time in between rests and naps. Chris hasn't been himself for a long time, even before all of this started to happen. He has been working very hard and feeling like he is not being appreciated nor respected at work. There is also talk that the company he works for is being sold, and as we all know there is always some truth to rumors.

I am worried for him, worried for me and for the kids. Will he be able to handle it all? Any man in his shoes would have a struggle ahead of him but that is not for me to worry about right now, it is surgery day and I have to go under the knife. I pray that two of the most important people in my life will be there with me holding each one of my hands.

We arrive at the hospital for 10:30am even though my surgery is not for a few more hours. We head for the registration desk with all of my necessary documents. After I register a nurse takes me to a room to prep me for surgery. Fortunately Chris is able to stay with me while the nurse hooks me up to an intravenous. It takes several attempts before the nurse is finally able to find a vein – the pain is excruciating for both me and Chris. I am finally able to rest comfortably in bed when Dr. Patel enters the room.

"Good morning Mr. and Mrs. Grice. How are we doing today?" he asks

"A little nervous, but I know this needs to be done." I respond.

"I understand, do you have any questions?"

"No, I don't think so"

Dr. Patel goes on to explain that my iron levels have dropped even further and he suggests that a blood transfusion is necessary. Apparently I am one of two of the worst cases that he has seen this year. Naturally I give my consent and the nurses continue to prepare me for surgery.

When they finally arrive to wheel me into the operating room I feel scared and emotional as I say my goodbyes to Chris. I can see that he is just as scared as I am. He takes my hand and walks with me as far as he can until he is told that he can go no further. He gives me a loving kiss on my forehead, tells me that he loves me and that he will be waiting for me as the doors close behind me.

The operating room is a busy place with the staff all a buzz. I am transferred onto the operating table and the anesthesiologist is waiting to administer the medication into my IV. I am feeling more and more relaxed. As I drift into a deep sleep, I can feel their presence and I know that all is going to be okay.

Chapter 5

A Mother's Life

Our Parents: Alfonso and Concetta

SHE WAS an attractive brunette with short styled hair. She took regular trips to the beauty parlor to get her hair set as many women her age did in the sixties. She wore no makeup except for her bright red lipstick. Her skin was so soft and milky and she had a Snow White look about her. She was a beautiful woman and she was my mother.

I have wonderful memories of mom, especially our regular trips downtown where we would go to Eaton's department store and admire the Window Displays at Christmas. We watched as a mechanical Santa and his elves made toys in the workshop and the figure skaters glided around on the make believe ice, while carolers sang our favorite songs. It was a magical time and I know that mom enjoyed it as much as I did.

I often think of her and ask myself whether she was truly happy? Did she ever really enjoy her life? It seemed at times like her life was one big chore after another and then she got cancer.

I was the youngest of three sisters and three brothers. Yes I was what you might say the accident in the family. My mom was forty two years old when she gave birth to me. She was so embarrassed to be pregnant because what it meant to the world was that she was "still doing it" at her age. In many ways, mom was a rather proper lady.

I remember dad telling me a story that mom went to see the family doctor, wondering how she could get around her unexpected pregnancy. Apparently, the family doctor had five sons and wanted a girl so badly, that he would take me off their hands if I were a girl. It was odd that dad would tell me such a thing.

But then he says "Once you were born, there was no way that mama could have ever given you up". I recall thinking, really?

Needless to say I grew up in the family I was born into. It was a very traditional Italian family; a Sicilian family to be precise. However, there are times when I have wondered what life would have been like as the only daughter of a doctor and five older brothers. Eventually, we found ourselves another family doctor. Despite hearing that hurtful story, I knew there was no way my mom could ever have given me up. My mother never in my whole life made me feel like I was unwanted or unloved. I knew I mattered to her and I knew that when the time came for her to die, that she did not want to leave me.

I forgave my mother for not wanting another child. She not only had five kids before me, but four other kids that did not survive. She had two sons die in Italy, her first born was a year old and the other was eighteen months. Then once she immigrated to Canada, she gave birth to twins; the girl was still born and the boy survived for only twenty-four hours. I can't even imagine the pain of losing a child. My mom went through a lot of hardship and a lot of pregnancies so after having all these kids, the thought of one more was likely more than she could bear. And what if something went wrong?

Then there was my dad. What was the real story there? There has been much speculation but it was really no secret that despite his good looks, blonde hair and blue eyes, it was not love at first sight for my mother. Apparently he was head over heels in love with her but as I grew older I could see that she didn't have that look in her eye. Their relationship was often conflicted and dad had a short fuse as they say. Even though we resented my dad for his quick temper, we knew that mom often knew which of his buttons to push and which ones not to push.

My father was the middle child of three and the oldest of the boys. He had a difficult life as an orphan. He would often tell us that he was taken in off the street by a relative when he was only eleven years old after his parents died. He would always say that he had a shovel in his hand early on in his life and worked to support his older sister and younger brother. My dad's father died when he was in his thirties after being bitten by a wild dog with rabies. His young mother was left to raise three children on her own. According to my mother, my grandmother was known as the town whore.

"She needed to support her children somehow". My mother would say.

She apparently contracted Venereal Disease and died. My father on the other hand, had his own version. His mother died mysteriously at the age of 33 from a rare blood disease. I often wonder if it wasn't VD, then what was this disease; cancer?

Like everyone else, dad just wanted someone to love him. My parents were from a very small town in Sicily called Racalmuto. It was the land of arranged marriages and in the 1937 my mother was nineteen years old when she married my father who was twenty-five. At that time she was considered a bit of an old maid. I don't understand why. She was an attractive woman from black and white pictures that I have seen. She had long braided dark brown hair and an olive complexion, even though I don't ever remember her having dark skin. It's almost as though she got lighter as she grew older.

Mom loved school and wanted to become a teacher. However that was not to be. Her mother apparently had other plans for her. I remember my mother telling the story to me and my sisters with a tear in her eye.

She would say "my teacher came to the house and begged my mother to let me go back to school." She told my mother "she is so smart she could be a teacher herself".

But no, her mother needed someone to clean the house and take care of her. My mother's dream died that day. I felt so bad for her. As a result she wanted us all to be school-teachers. Although we are all teachers of something in this world, that role was only to be filled by my sister, Tina, the oldest of the girls. I guess my mother learned at an early age that her role was to serve others, get married, and have ten kids and that is what she did. Overall, she was a good mother to us. I know she had her favorites; fortunately I was one of them. Parents always say they love their children all the same. That is such bull, or at least it was in my family. My dad had his favorites too, but I most definitely wasn't one of them.

I was fourteen years old when my mom went in for a routine hernia operation. She had never been in the hospital as long as I was around. After all I was the last baby. So it seemed strange not to have her around the house. I was missing her and I hoped she would be coming home soon. I remember going to the hospital to see her. I was so excited and nervous because I did not really know what to expect. And anyways, I don't even think I had been in a hospital before then. My candy striping days with my best friend Cecilia happened the summer after. So I was feeling a little uneasy and uncomfortable seeing my mother lying in a hospital bed. I do not remember what we said or even how she looked. I just remember thinking that I wanted her to come home. What I did not know at that time was that my life would be forever changed when she did.

In the meantime, we waited while doctors and nurses came in and out to check my mom and speak with my family. I was not really sure what was going on at the time. At the far end of the hallway there were two chairs just under what looked like a window sill. Just below the window sill there was a small table with a statue of the Virgin Mary. There are a lot of them around in Catholic hospitals especially in those days. My sisters and I went for a walk and landed at the end of the hall by the Virgin Mary's statue. My sisters at that time were twenty one and twenty two years old. I could see by their faces that they had something very important to tell me. I never would have guessed what it was. I remember them telling me that when mom had the hernia operation the doctors found this thing called cancer in her body. Back in 1976 cancer was in fact this thing that nobody really knew much about. At least we didn't. All we really knew was that if you got it, you died from it. And that is what my family was told. Apparently, my mom had one month to live. I remember the three of us cried in each other's arms. How could this be happening to her and to our family? She was fifty six years old.

I was only fourteen years old, had just started high school and was at the peak of my selfishness. I remember thinking that I still needed my mother. We all did. I wondered what my life would be like without her around. My sisters, I am sure were thinking the same thing. They were older than me but let's face it, at what age do you stop needing a mother? When I think back on it now, I know that we were all in shock. We were afraid of what all this would mean for our family. I remember that my sisters and I held each other and cried in front of the Virgin Mary's statue. After awhile, we dried up our tears and never spoke of this thing called cancer again.

Chapter 6

Breathing A Sigh of Relief

THE BEST part of having surgery is when you are in the recovery room resting comfortably under those warm blankets. I feel safe and protected and want this feeling to last a little bit longer but then I realize as I am coming out of it, that I can't even wiggle my little toe without pressing the pain pump. I am in the recovery room for longer than expected. The surgery was longer than anticipated as well due to a complication. I do have all the luck don't I? Actually I am very lucky. Apparently the lining of my uterus had become so thick that it attached itself to my bowel. Having to remove my uterus and the thickened lining was rather tricky so as to not damage or puncture my bowel. After all, I no longer need my uterus, but my bowel is a different story. In order to access this area, the laparoscopic incision that was planned, was not enough. The long and the short of it is that I have a huge scar from east to west. The good news is that you can't really see it because of the overhang of my belly. All joking aside I am a new woman now. I have new blood and way more than they even expected. Because of the complication, I lost a lot of blood and additional units were needed. The best thing of all is that I am not bleeding anymore. I also had a bladder repair while I was under. Surgical complications and all, I have a whole new life ahead of me. I am free of all my horrible thoughts and tragic scenarios that I envisioned in my mind, and free to live the life that for a brief time was threatened by the thought of Cancer. So much in my life will change.

The porter wheels me back me up to my room and I feel that comatose feeling again. I can hear voices around me but I can't move my body. I can hear Chris's soft and gentle voice and feel his love just by his soothing tone. I know that I am alive and that my family is here. I also hear my sister Tina's voice. I knew she would be here to ensure that I would come out of surgery alive. My brother in law Rocky is also here. His voice is very strong and carries well. I am sure that the whole surgical ward can hear him too. He doesn't like hospitals much and I am sure he came because my sister does not like to drive downtown.

Rocky has known me since I was eleven years old playing intramural basketball. He reminds me often that we never won a game. Despite that, I am most grateful to Rock for getting me through high school math with at least a passing grade. Our whole family still is mathematically challenged.

Last but certainly not least, my brother John and his wife Cynthia are here. The two of them travel by bus everywhere despite having physical challenges that make walking painful. I am very happy that they have come to see me in the hospital. My brother John is such a kind and patient man. I think back to when I was young and he would take me to all the fun places like the circus and the park. In many ways, I think that he was my best friend in those early days and I know that he had as much fun as I did.

I open my eyes and see my husband hovering over me and smiling as though he really thought he'd never see me again. I am so relieved to see him too. We have been through so much together over the years. Throughout the evening

27

there are other family and friends that come to see me. It is wonderful to be surrounded by all that love and support. I am told that because of the bowel complication, the additional units of blood from the transfusion, and the huge scar, that my risk of infection is greater. So I have to stay for an extra night.

My children will come to see me on my second night of my hospital stay. I miss them. Hopefully by then, I will be up and about. For now I lay down in pain, administering my own dosage of Oxycontin. Imagine. But the night time comes and everyone goes home and there we are me and Josephine.

Chapter 7

Me and Josephine

YOU DON'T often hear the name Josephine as much these days, so I get rather excited on those rare occasions. You can imagine my surprise when who should be laying in the bed next to me? A little old lady named Josephine. I am told that she is about ninety one years old and she is so tiny and frail. I don't really know the extent of her problems but I hear that she has horrible bed sores. The nursing staff is trying to keep her comfortable and I have seen a lot of family around her. She has one niece in particular that is often at the hospital for long periods of time. I think to myself "How nice is that. Josephine was obviously good to them and now they are returning the favor". I don't think she has any children of her own.

All of my family and friends have left. The night has come for Josephine too and everyone in her camp has gone home. I am still feeling groggy but I hear a little voice say, "Is anybody out there?" All is quiet. I don't know who she is talking to.

Again, I hear "Is anybody out there?" A small smile comes to me as I remember that being the title of one of Alice Cooper's songs or albums in the seventies. But the voice is sounding more distressed.

I answer "Yes Josephine I am here"

In her old and frail voice she says "I hate to be a bother dear, but I need a nurse"

"No problem Josephine" and I push the red button. Needless to say this continues through most of the night.

Now into my second evening, the situation is even worse. It's to the point that I am roaming the halls just to get out of the room. It is good for me to walk even though it is 2 am. The nurses are very proud of my progress and actually so am I. I figure recovery isn't going to be as bad as I anticipated. The nurses however are trying to find me another room so I can get some sleep but I decline the opportunity. If I am to be honest, I am happy to have Josephine in my room. I just love saying her name again and again. It makes me feel even closer to my own Josephine.

Chapter 8

My Own Josephine

MY JOSEPHINE goes by the name Josie. Josie is the second youngest in the family and the middle child of the last three girls. She is seven years older than me and one year younger than my oldest sister Tina. Certainly because of the age difference, my sisters were very close growing up and shared pretty much everything. I was always the loner, never really having anyone in the family I could hang out with. When I was a baby, I was a wonderful addition to the family. Who needed pretend dolls when they had a real live one in me? But once that wore off and mom was asking for extra help, it wasn't so great after all. Taking part in my care was something that my oldest sister, Tina embraced at the time. But I think that in some ways, she later became very resentful. I can't really blame her. Just because she was the oldest, it didn't mean that she always needed to be more responsible. I think she may have felt that she missed out on her childhood. To this day I think that role still affects our relationship because Tina is still very motherly toward me. But Josie was content to play her games outside, banging her sock and ball against the brick wall of our house. She loved to skip and from a young age she had a sense of fun to her.

Josie was such a pretty girl. She stood at an average height of five two and had the peaches and cream complexion that other girls would die for. She had hazel eyes that turned green sometimes depending on how the light hit her. She had light brown hair with an auburn tone to it. Her hair was always on the frizzy side and she hated that. But that was before low lights and hi lights, relaxers and all the hair products we have now. She was beautiful, but it was her inner beauty that really shined. She was a loving daughter, a caring sister, a loyal wife and an outstanding mother. She had a big heart and big dreams.

Unlike me and my other sister, Josie did not attend university even though she often received better marks than us. Josie had other plans for her life and took a different path. Josie wanted to put her keen organizational skills and pleasant manner to good use and decided that she wanted to become a secretary, better known now as an administrative assistant. She intended to go to college but came across an opportunity to work for our brother, Joe who was in business for himself at the time. She was very happy for a while but hard times fell onto my brother's business and that meant no paycheck for Josie. This seemed to set the path for financial hardship that would haunt Josie for much of her adult life.

I remember her going out on a few dates and I mean a few. My parents were very traditional Italians and that meant that they were not in favor of the dating scene. At some point they caught on and realized, that is how you meet the person that could potentially be your husband. Then the big night came when she met the guy she knew she would marry. John was a sweetheart and he had all the right moves and knew all the right things to say to impress a rather sheltered Italian girl. And anyways he spoke Italian and worked in a law firm as a clerk. My mom thought he was a lawyer, or wait, did he tell my sister he was a lawyer to impress her? Whatever it was she was head over heels in love with him and so was my mother.

It was not a long engagement but my sister went through her fair share of frustration as he was always late and kept her waiting. John was a little laid back and although this was a quality my sister tolerated, I think his suaveness was part of his appeal. She was prompt and organized but could get herself really worked up. Who knew back then that his procrastination would lead to a lot of aggravation in the future?

I was really close to John at the time and we would sit for long periods of time talking. He was great at giving advice about love, friendship and relationships. Honestly he was like another brother to me. John was a handsome guy with light brown wavy hair that was receding. You knew the hair wasn't going to last forever. He was very charming and charismatic and had a beautiful smile that showed his warm and caring personality. I could see why Josie was drawn to him.

John and Josie married and they became the couple everyone included. They were both such nice people. John had a very large network of friends who welcomed Josie in their circle. At the time she was working for a large company and was doing well until the company was sold and moved to the States. After four years of marriage, Josie found herself without a job so it seemed like a good time to start a family. Josie always wanted to be a stay at home mother. I remember mom being furious with her. She felt that Josie had not waited long enough and ruined her life by getting pregnant. I have to say that was terrible of my mother, but look where she was coming from; nine pregnancies, four baby deaths and a lot of broken dreams and missed opportunities. We were all very happy for John and Josie and my mother, well she came around. Six weeks later, my other sister, Tina announced that she was pregnant too. Oh my poor mother. She didn't get to see either of the babies. She died in September 1981 while my sisters were pregnant. That marked the beginning of a trend in our family.

John and Josie had a beautiful baby boy named Anthony. My sister insisted that his name not be abbreviated. Her beautiful angel boy was never to be referred to or called Tony. Anthony was a real heavyweight at birth weighing 9lb 3 oz. No one was more surprised about this than Josie and she often joked about the size of Anthony's head. Anthony had the chubbiest cheeks and the cutest curl on his lip every time he smiled which was often. Anthony was the happiest baby I had ever seen. Needless to say it took Josie some time to recuperate.

Two years later Paul arrived. Talk about a cherub! Paul had the dreamiest blue eyes, the blondest hair and the widest smile. Paul was so cute that if we dressed him in pink and threw on a bonnet, he could pass for a little girl. Josie loved her boys. They were both so beautiful and so gentle but she longed for a daughter. Mothers and sons often share a very close bond and Josie and her boys were no different. But some mothers, whether openly or secretively, wish for a daughter as well. Josie often joked about how fertile she was so we knew that a third pregnancy was in her future.

They had a small back split which Josie thought would be a good starter home and anyways it was in their budget. Interest rates were at an all time high in the eighties. It was the coziest house that Josie decorated with her style and good taste. The rooms were small and comfortable. There was no eat- in kitchen so the dining room table was where it all happened. It had three bedrooms with the boys sharing a room. There was just a warm comforting feeling when you walked through the front door. No foyer. You walked in and one step to the right you were in the living room and one step forward you were in the kitchen where there was always something baking. If it wasn't her bacon and cheddar biscuits it was her banana bread or shortbread. My personal favorite was her chocolate chip cookies. Oh the list goes on and on. Everything she baked was golden. This was a perfect example of a young family who loved and cared for one another and understood the value of what they had. That is often rare and Josie knew that. But there was something missing and she knew that too. She wanted more and thought she deserved more.

John at the time was self employed. He had not always been in business for himself. He worked for a lawyer but unfortunately the lawyer died suddenly. John was out of a job so he decided to continue to do what he was doing and be his own boss. Initially it sounded like a good idea but there were a few problems. John took his time with everything and well, did not always demand payment when payment was due. This used to drive Josie crazy. She managed the money but when there is little money to manage, the stress builds and builds and builds. Where does all this stress go?

Financial worries continued to be a burden with Josie doing a lot of the worrying. I'm sure in his own way John did too. But it was different for him he was working but Josie was at home with the boys. Where could she go? How could she leave them? Who could she leave them with? We did not have our mother and both my sister Tina and I had careers and worked full time. All these questions and more worries. It is not easy running a household and raising two kids on a limited budget. She did not want her children to go without and as hard as it was for Josie to leave her children, she returned to the workforce. She made arrangements with John's mother to care for the boys and took a job. It was a good one and it paid well too. It seemed to help them out considerably. Josie enjoyed the fact that they were slowly moving toward financial freedom and the burden was slowly lifting, but she hated to leave the boys. She was still longing for a daughter and became pregnant with Andrea. One could only predict that she would be a beauty, and she was. Andrea was our very own version of Goldie Locks. Josie's family was now complete. Tina and I were so pissed with her decision to not return to work. There was such a thing as maternity leave and a lot of women took them. Tina had already taken two leaves for both her little boys. But that was not what Josie wanted. She loved being a homemaker. She loved being a mother. She was great at doing both. She wanted to be home with her three babies. I guess she knew something that we didn't.

Chapter 9

The Little Sister

I GREW UP very much on my own. Being so much younger than all my siblings, I had little in common and to be quite honest, I'm sure I was the pain in the ass little sister. My sisters were four days short of being one year apart from each other which meant they went to school together and had a lot of the same friends. They also shared a room together forever. They argued about stuff that sisters that close usually complain about. As young girls I remember the arguments "Move over you're hogging all the sheets" or "Who just farted?" That was usually my oldest sister, Tina. To this day she continues to suffer with gastric issues. There were times of course when they would both gang up on me and say that I was an accident and mom and dad didn't want me. I would be reduced to tears and I didn't even know about my mom's plan to get around the pregnancy with the doc who had five sons.

I had very different relationships with both my sisters. It's funny how my oldest sister was the one who helped my mother with my care, but I never felt nurtured by her at that time. Honestly, as I have grown older I have come to appreciate my sister's nurturing qualities. It was not always this way and it was not always easy for we are both very strong and outspoken. Getting along with Josie was always so easy. She never yelled at me or let it been known that she was the older sister. When I was in high school and needed to buy a Christmas gift for a boyfriend my parents never knew I had, it was Josie that gave me the money to buy it. She was always so patient and understanding. I'm not really sure how our relationship evolved or when we really got close. Thinking back it may have been after our mother died.

My mom's funeral was in September and coincided with frosh week at the university. I was just starting my first year and obviously missed the first week of parties and other festivities. Not much into it anyways, but by March of that school year my sister had Anthony. The following year Josie was still at home with Anthony and was able to type all my essays and papers that were due. Yes, there were no computers in those days. I remember we would put the kettle on and I would dictate the essay to her and she would type it as I read it out. We both liked the pressure because the papers were due either that same day or the next. Anthony was either asleep or playing amongst us while we worked. He was such a good baby. I don't think he ever went through the terrible twos.

Our relationship just grew from there. Paul was born a few years later. What a beauty he was but he had a little more spunk to him. Josie was a busy lady but she always made time for me. I was so fortunate that she had such patience for me and all my stories, all my dilemmas and so much drama as we say now. We drank so much tea and could chat for hours. Every now and then I would think that it was so selfish of me to take up so much of her time. She had children to take care of and they needed her attention. Mind you, it's not like they were ever neglected. We were always where they were. But whenever my guilt set in, Josie would laugh and say "Don't be so ridiculous. You keep me young and connected to the outside world". I would think really? I didn't understand that until years later when I too became a stay at home mom like Josie.

She made it all look so easy. I remember her getting so upset when working mothers would say how nice it must be to be a stay at home mother. Josie would respond "It has it's perks" with a pleasant, but yet snarky tone. I knew what she was really thinking and how much she was sacrificing. Limited shopping sprees and few family vacations. My oldest sister had a career and worked full time. She helped out a lot and often bought the boys clothes. She had two beautiful boys herself so what she bought for hers she bought for Josie's boys as well. Although it was appreciated, it was often hard for Josie to accept. "Nobody likes to feel like charity" she would often say to me.

Worrying about not having enough money was always in Josie's thoughts. Your outlook on life, the way you feel about yourself and how you view the world. is all affected by the amount of money in your wallet. They say money isn't everything and that is true. But it sure makes life a little easier.

Josie and I would talk for hours about what our lives would be like if we had a lot of money. The freedom we thought we would have. We thought that if we had an abundance of money we wouldn't have much to worry about. Wow! Were we ever wrong.

Chapter 10

Is History Repeating Itself?

I THINK BACK to when this whole nightmare started. I was not keeping a journal at the time but I remember every moment and every feeling as though it had just happened. Josie was experiencing some discomfort and because I was the queen of indigestion, she came to me for some advice. She would often feel full very quickly without eating much so I suggested the usual suckable tablets. However, none of these temporary solutions really offered her any relief, so she decided to book an appointment with the family doctor.

Josie was never a big eater and usually tried to eat the right foods. Sure she loved her salt and her sugary snacks but it was all in moderation. The doctor decided to perform a series of tests and ultrasounds to help determine the problem. Initially it looked like it was a virus or an infection of some sort. So she was prescribed some antibiotics. Back in 1994, getting a prescription for antibiotics was a lot easier than it is now. An ulcer perhaps would not be surprising, given the fact that Josie worried about everyone and everything. However, this infection was not clearing up and that led doctors to believe that perhaps they were not on the right track.

Several months later, more tests and weeks of waiting for
results took us to May. Finally Josie had an appointment with
the family doctor. I offered to take Josie for her appointment
and waited patiently while she went into the examination
room. I remember feeling a little restless and worried wondering what the outcome of this visit would be. It felt like I
had been waiting forever when suddenly Josie came through
the waiting area. She quickly looked into my eyes and then
walked right out the door as if she didn't see me. I felt a quick
flutter in my stomach as I followed her outside and we both
walked toward my car. Neither of us said a word until I finally
asked, "What did the doctor say?" At that moment, I was not
so sure that I really wanted to know. She did not answer me.
I thought to myself "Is there something she doesn't want me
to know?"

It was a really hot day in May and when we got into the
car, I had to open the windows to let out some of the heat.
"What were the test results, Jos?" I asked with more asser-
tion. I could see that she was hesitating and avoiding eye
contact when she slowly raised her head and looked at me.
We both looked into each other's eyes and I could see that
Josie had a look of shock and disbelief. I didn't know what to
say or do.

Then she quietly whispered "You are not going to believe
this but it's our worst nightmare".

I looked back at her and before I could tell her what I was
thinking, I heard Josie say with a quiver, "I have cancer."

I sat there in shock wondering if the words were coming
out of her mouth or from some other planet. It didn't feel
real but yet I knew it was. For once in my life I couldn't find
the words to express how I felt. We stared into each other's
eyes and cried our hearts out. I had no idea how much time
had passed, but we knew that we couldn't hide in the car
forever. So we dried up our tears and drove home to her

house to put the kettle on.

This was all too familiar and I couldn't help but think to myself that history was repeated itself.

It was really only fourteen years ago when mom died of cancer. We all had a hard time. Even though dad was the dominant one, we all knew that mom ran the show and kept it all going. Our mother was a stay at home mom too. She went to work at the cotton mill factory but after one day came home in tears and told my father that there was no way that she could ever go back. She promised my father that from that day on, she would do whatever was necessary to economize. From what I have been told, she did not get any opposition from dad and so it began. In mom's effort to economize, she baked bread and cookies daily and made everything from scratch. It was all good stuff, but when you are a kid, you want the bought cookies and sliced bread like some of the English kids had.

When mom died we had not ever known anyone that had died before. So it sucked that our first experience with death was our own mother. My sisters were both expecting babies, and my brothers, despite being older and two of them had been married for years, they kept regular contact with mom especially my brother Sam.

She loved her middle boy Sammy. They spoke on the phone almost daily and in the early days when Sammy had first gotten married; he would come over for lunch before going off to work the afternoon shift. Mom would have a huge sirloin round steak ready for him to devour and they would talk. About what, I have no idea. I recently shared this fond memory with my sister in law, Angie, who after all these years had no knowledge of Sam's regular pit stop. I guess it was their little secret. Sammy had a quick temper and piercing blue eyes and was somewhat of a lady's man in his youth. He would give you the shirt off his back and was always there to lend a hand to whoever was in need. He was definitely one of mom's favorites but then again so was Johnny.

He was her other blonde hair blue eyed boy. We all knew that John was the best baby of all with his mild temperament and easy going personality. His good natured personality continued well into adulthood. John was the last to marry of the boys. In fact both my sisters married before John. He was always a late bloomer and definitely beat to the rhythm of his own drum. I suppose all those years in a band gave him a lot of practice. John actually was a drummer in a rock band called 007. In the sixties they played at all the weddings and other social events. I remember as a little girl, all the band members would gather together at our house for band practice and my mom would make homemade pizza of course for all the boys. I was about four years old and I remember sitting on my brother's lap as he played the drums. Those were good times.

My oldest brother Joe was in a band too. They were called the Gold Tones and they played more than the local Italian weddings and dances. They had actual gigs outside the city and even went to Alaska. There was even talk of record deals and contracts but outside pressures like girlfriends, parents and education brought the boys on separate paths. It was amazing how two of my three brothers played in bands and neither of them had any lessons. We have always been a musical family. Dad loved to dance and mom apparently loved to sing.

My brother Joe seems to have some of the best memories of my mom. He was her first surviving child and since mom was young at the time, Joe remembers mom to be a very playful mother. Back in Italy where all three of my brothers were born, there was not really that much to do but play li rocci which is really our modern day jacks. Joe and mom would play for hours until mom would panic because it would soon be time for dad to come home and she needed to prepare dinner. I love talking to my brother Joe about the history of the family. He is the only one who remembers our grandparents and our parents in the very early days. In his own way, Joe too had a special relationship with our mother.

Chapter 11

What Is It About Mothers?

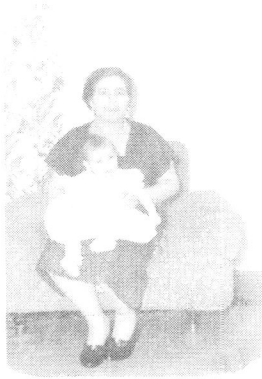

My mother and I

NO REALLY. You've got to ask yourself, what is so special about having a mother? I suppose the answer to that question is very different depending on who you ask. I know some people who have major mommy issues and others who cannot make a decision without their mother's input. Then again there are others like me who don't have a choice and go through life making their own decisions secretly wondering if their mother would approve. But what makes many of us call for our mothers when we are sick or cry our hearts out when our heart has been broken? Why is it that we long for our mothers when they have died or feel anger toward them when we feel that they have abandoned us?

Despite the uniqueness of our relationships with our mothers, one thing is for sure. We can all agree for the most part that we expect our mother to care for us and comfort us and we depend on them when there is no one else in the world that we can turn to. A mother is not only someone who cooks, cleans and makes sure we have clean clothes to wear, but we rely on her to nurture us, praises us and encourages us. She can even get away with a little white lie so as to not hurt our feelings. I remember asking my mother so many times, "Mom does my bum look big in these jeans"?

My mother would always reply, "no mama, you looka beautiful, no worry". I knew she wasn't being completely honest with me, but it was what I needed to hear and she knew that. That is not to say that mom never passed judgment or let me know of her expectations. I can recall many times my mom reminding my sisters and I to keep those legs closed and not even think of coming home pregnant. I used to think that she was so obsessed with those thoughts. But I was her baby and I knew what that role represented. Despite the arduous task of raising all of her children, I knew my mom loved us and was there for us all.

Josie was no exception. She took her mothering role seriously. Her children always came first and it was her goal in life to ensure that she raised children who were good, kind and caring people. Sure she did the usual mom thing and cooked and cleaned and baked. She was a great baker and started to make novelty cakes for birthdays. The kids loved their Sesame Street and Disney character cakes. She even made me a beautiful Donald Duck cake for my thirtieth birthday. She always put so much love and time into each of her creations. She was a very detailed person and it was her attention to the little things that made her special. She always put the fun into things. She was never intimidating and her understanding nature made it easy for the kids to fess up when they had been up to no good. She would often take on all the kids during the P.D days and have Tina's boys Michael and Mathew join her kids for a day of fun. They adored their auntie Josie too.

She knew that she was making a financial sacrifice by being a stay at home mom. But despite the constant worry and stress, it was worth it to her. She was always at the bus stop to pick up the kids after school. She would give her full attention to them and listen to their stories about the day's events and always be ready to offer praise and encouragement. Her fridge always displayed the latest masterpieces. She shared her praise with all three, but always gave that little something extra for Paul's artistic talents, Anthony's creative ideas and Andrea's helpful nature. She was always preparing baked goods for the children to share with their classmates. Josie chose her role as a homemaker and mother and she chose it with pride.

Of all the pots of tea and cookies and conversations we have had over the years, there was always so much to talk about. Now, it all came down to this. Josie received her diagnosis and we honestly didn't know what to say. We stared a lot at each other with her beautiful hazel eyes and my big brown eyes, we communicated without words. Oh my God. At that point there were few tears. I think just shock. She was thirty-eight years old with a husband and three beautiful children; eleven, nine and six. There was a sadness that no words could describe. Josie needed to call John who was at work.

Then she thought, "I got to call Tina and dad. Oh my God how do we give this news to dad and my kids, my beautiful kids" and at that thought, Josie's tears began to roll down her face.

I did what every good sister would do and assured Josie that there was no way that this disease would take her over. She was young and healthy and that this whole thing was somehow just unreal. Josie agreed and made her phone calls and I made myself available to the children when they got home from school. . The following months were a blur as Josie shared the devastating news with family and friends. Our chins up days were short lived and we had plenty of up and down days. We were feeling such disbelief and shock. We cried and cried and cried. More tests and more waiting was more than anyone could bear especially Josie who worried about everything by nature, really had something to worry about now. She knew that she was in for the fight of her life and that is what she did.

Chapter 12

The Power of The Written Word

THERE IS a lot to be said about the written word. I mentioned earlier that we are not a mathematical family. Instead we are a family of thinkers, readers and writers. And it all started with mom who took great pride in her ability to read and write. I have fond memories of my mother sitting at the dining room table, a gift that she had purchased for my father on his birthday, writing letters to her half siblings in Italy and in Belgium. It is amazing the things we remember when we are children, like the envelopes with the air mail stamps and the thin writing pad where she would write all of her thoughts in Italian. I recently found letters that she had received from her siblings in the 50's. In reading them, I could almost hear the dialogue in my head.

There is something so powerful about the written word. There is a certain validation that occurs when we put our feelings down on paper. There is a truth about who we are and what we believe based on how we feel. Our writings often capture our raw emotions of whatever situation we find ourselves writing about at that time. Letter writing seemed to be a ritual for my mother. I remember she would set aside some time in the afternoon, and retrieve her letter writing supplies from the side table drawer of that same dining room set that she purchased for dad and write. It seemed as though it was her time to reconnect with her loved ones who were far but it was also something she did for herself. And as I grew older I understood the importance of that time.

Although I have no relatives abroad that I can write to , my journal became my ritual and my time to escape from my life, reconnect with myself and express my raw emotions about my life and what was going on in it. My journals have recorded some of my most personal and challenging experiences in my life and when I go back and read through them, it often gives me hope that if I can get through that, I can get through anything. I am not sure what will become of all of my journals. I hope that my children may find them of interest someday and perhaps see another side of me. A side that portrays me not only as their mother, but a person who had dreams, insecurities and fears, not to mention my share of disappointments. Many of which I have overcome and others that still remain a challenge. It would be my gift, my legacy to my children. So I had hoped that when Josie decided to write in her journal, she too would leave a legacy for her children. She too would share her most personal battle with this disease and show a side of herself to her kids about what it was like for her, not to mention how she felt about them. It was shocking for me to read the pages of Josie's journal and not read any of that. Although I read about how she spent her days and all the things that she did in a day, I think my God what strength. But I also feel the emptiness and the void of emotion in many of those pages.

No matter how many times I read Josie's journal I cry. She must have been so terrified. It's been nearly eighteen years and it brings me right back to the last year that we spent with her. I look at her hand writing and read her words. It's almost as though she is talking in my ear. I swear sometimes I feel her so near.

On August 16th 1994, Josie wrote in her
journal for the first time:

It's been suggested to me that I write down my thoughts
to express my frustration and relieve stress. I thought I knew
what frustration and stress was all about but I was wrong.
Discovering that you have a dreaded disease is the true
meaning of stress. Cancer was always the scariest word I
knew. Now it was to become my whole life.

My discomfort started at Christmas 1993, feeling very full
without eating much. I had lost 36 lbs on weight watchers
two years prior and felt great about myself at 125lbs. Maybe
I should have been more cautious about my eating habits.
Some days I ate very little but had a ton of energy. Running
around with the kids, working at the school and taking care
of dad's needs didn't leave much time for a good sit down
breakfast and lunch. Anyways whatever it was my stomach
was not right anymore. It rumbled from hunger but felt so
strange it vibrated to the touch. March and April became
difficult to eat anything without that sharp pain between my
breasts. At first it felt like my heart. In April I went to see
Dr. Z who immediately started to treat me for ulcers. Two
weeks later no change so he sent me for a barium swallow
x-ray. They found something because I barely arrived home
and Dr. Z had called to arrange an endoscopy with Dr. Y, a
cancer specialist. That was Thursday May 8 I think. That was
a painful experience I thought I was going to choke. But I
didn't. They took a biopsy of what was in my stomach. Later
Dr. Z told me it appeared to be gastric lymphoma. I almost
didn't hear what he said. I was stunned and foggy headed. But
I know I was in for the worst battle of my life. Sal took me to
the doctor thank God. I blurted out cancer and we both cried

like babies. The days after were blurry and all I know was an appointment was set up to see Dr. C, a surgeon. He scheduled surgery for June 16/94. Much to his shock, he had to remove my entire stomach not the half that they had thought before. I also lost my spleen and gallbladder because I had stones. Three surgeries in one . What a joke! Recovery was very slow, My hospital stay was only one week. While there I met two people Dr. F and his assistant Susan. They give me all these statistics but I'm in a daze. All I hear is that this cancer usually comes back 50/50. What odds. They talk of chemo and radiation or possibly no treatment at all. What should I do? I must take all precautions to save my life. Therapy will increase the chances they say. My chemo was to start July 11 /94. In the meantime I am recovering from the surgery. It's a long haul. Food is not appealing. I get the heaves often and I feel nauseated all the time. And I have diarrhea regularly. I am down to 116lbs. They decided to delay my chemo to July 18/94 another joke! Happy birthday to me. Overall the week was fine until Friday. My mouth is full of cankers and sores and I had diarrhea .They both lasted until the next Friday. I used medication for the nausea and diarrhea but it didn't help too much. I should have taken the full dose but I didn't. Now for my herbal strategy! I'm taking taheebo or pan'arco tea on the advice from the author and cancer survivor Josif who I met and purchased the teas from. He swears by it, but strongly condemns chemo and radiation. I have been taking the tea daily 4 cups, and then I hear from Sal of a new herbal mix called Essiac. I read all the books about Rene Caisse the originator of the mix. It's a blood strengthener and she has claimed that it has cured cancer patients of all kinds. My connection for this tea is a cancer survivor Mary C and today I picked up my first case at a cost of $200.00. Dad was kind enough to give me the amount. Mary gave me hers to tide me over until the shipment arrives. She is such a kind lady.

Today she received her own packages and will be making her own tea from now on and will show me next month how to do it. Chemo started again yesterday August 15th/94 another joke, mom's birthday. I feel a little tired today and my recent good appetite since taking Essiac is gone again. Today I am just tired and pms cranky. Bye for now. I 'm taking my tea and going to bed.

Chapter 13

Let's Just Pretend.....

IT IS really hard to find the words to describe what it is like to see a young beautiful and gentle woman go through what Josie was dealing with. It all happened so fast that none of us really knew for sure if this was really happening. I remember waking up each morning and thinking, please God tell me that this was one horrifying nightmare. Let's just go back to the way life used to be because ... and anyways our lives were not really all that bad. It had been about fourteen years since we lost mom and although there are many times when we still long for mom, we have learned to live without her in our lives. That has not been easy. I pleaded with God or whoever else was listening, not to take another one of our family members away from us. Our feelings were a mixture of disbelief, anger, and sadness. We were scared to death ourselves. We knew what she was up against. We had already lived it and we knew all about the deterioration that comes along with having cancer. There was no way that this was going to happen and to our Josie, no way. My oldest brother Joe started to investigate many of the naturalist clinics outside of Canada that claimed to have saved the lives of many. There was a cost involved and the resources were being offered. But it was not to be.

I remember the day we had the consultation with the doctors. We were all sitting around a table in this room when Josie learned that she had a 50/50 chance of survival. They told us that the type of cancer that she had was aggressive and spreads like wildfire. It was a stomach cancer called linitus plastica. They explained that it was not a tumor but a sheet of cancer that spread and attached itself over her organs like a piece of saran wrap. It was a rare form particularly in someone as young as Josie. Her prognosis was bleak and they did not feel that she could survive past ten months. OH MY GOD! We were stunned. What happened to the 50/50? I remember looking at Josie and she looked right through me. I knew she was numb. She had just received a death sentence for something that she had never done or deserved. We said nothing in that meeting. There was nothing to say and no words could ever express our deepest fear and sadness for what we were now facing. "Ten months is less than a year. It is a little over six months and only two seasons out of four". My mind was racing. This can't be happening. I have always considered myself to be a person who wants to be in the know so that I can prepare myself for what I think is to come. But in this situation, I knew that nothing was going to prepare me for what was to come; and Josie? I honestly think that she was thinking that they were talking about someone else.

I remember going to the hospital one morning after her first surgery, and there she was propped up in her bed putting on the finishing touches and adding some gloss to her already full lips. I asked her what was going on and she told me in a very cheerful voice that she talked her doctor into letting her go home. She was being discharged today. She asked me to help her get her things together and that John was on his way. She was ready to go home and as strange as it sounded, it almost felt that she was no longer sick. It seemed as though everything was going to be okay. As confused as I was, I decided to go along with this. After all I could pretend that this was one big misunderstanding. I was perfectly fine to live in denial for as long as we could.

Chapter 14

The Tea of Life

August 17th 1994 Josie wrote:

> Third day of chemo is over. Marney came this morning and Sara drove me home. I don't feel too bad just a little tired by this evening. I'm sipping my essiac and going to bed. Good night.

I remember when we discovered this Essiac. I was sure that this was going to be what saved her life. It made a lot of sense as it saved the lives of so many people. It really gave Josie and all of us hope that she had a fighting chance. It meant that there really was an end to this horrific situation and we could all just go back to our lives with the knowledge of how precious life can be. But our lives were forever changed and there was no turning back. Our prayers were filled with hope that a miracle would happen and that our beautiful Josie would live a life free of cancer, watching her children grow. But that horrifying fear would always creep its way into our thoughts and bring us to tears as we imagined what our lives would be like without her.

August 18th /94 Josie wrote:

Fourth day and feeling very tired. I slept this afternoon. Tina came for the day. I felt nauseated several times today. Tonight I am so tired I can't stand. I'll call it a night very early.

August 19th/94 Josie wrote:

Last day of chemo for this month and I am a little tired not as much as yesterday, with only one bout of diarrhea. Chiara was here for the day and Tina came later with the kids. We chatted the whole day. The Aqua fine rep came tonight for a demo. I'm sure we will go for it. It is worth any amount to keep the water drinkable for my family. Good night.

Chapter 15

Touched by Spirit

August 20/94 Josie wrote:

Today is tomato day at dad's house. The guys went last night to get a good start and all was done today. I even went and put my two cents worth. Dad was happy to see me. I enjoy watching the husbands John, Rock, Chris, and brother John listening and being so tolerant of dad when he is uptight. We were home by 8:00pm and I began to read and finished Embraced by the light. I found it so easy to absorb. What an enlightening book. I feel that everything I learned as a child was verified. I began to doubt the existence of God, heaven and angels. Now I feel that what I have learned then has been truly acknowledged by someone.

August 21/94 Josie wrote:

Last night as I slept I felt a hand touch my shoulder 3 times like a gentle pat. It woke me, I thought it was John but he was asleep.

I felt scared and confused but fell right back to sleep. I prayed to my guardian angels that night so sincerely, maybe it let me know I was heard. My chemo symptoms are sort of lingering, this morning I have a touch of diarrhea and a slight sore on the bottom of my lip, only once nausea. Next month I will have no symptoms at ALL! After church and after pancake lunch, we went to dads to put away tomato jars. Dad was a little testy and Tina got angry with him.

Chapter 16

The Infamous Tomato Weekend

OH YES the tomato weekend. How can we forget those days when everything else stopped? You didn't dare make any other plans on that sacred weekend. Every Italian kid growing up knows that it's a big deal. In the early days it was a trip to the farm because "that is where you gotta the best tomatoes for the best price". Dad used to say.

He would always try to grab a few extra tomatoes and throw them around in the trunk of the car so that they looked like the bushels had spilled over. Yes I said bushels usually about fifteen of them full to the brim, plus the extra spillage. Dad was always so pumped. You could see that he was getting excited but along with that excitement was the anxiety that would nearly always lead to some angry outburst during the infamous tomato weekend.

Eventually a quick trip to the grocery store was more convenient. Those were sad days for my husband who enjoyed the farm experience. In fact Chris enjoyed the whole tomato weekend. Growing up as an only child in an English and French Canadian family, whose parents had divorced when he was thirteen, he enjoyed any opportunity that brought the family together. And fortunately in our family, there were many of them.

We were always a close family and enjoyed each other's company. Both Tina and Josie's boys were the same age. Michael was born six weeks after Anthony and Matthew was two years younger than Paul. The boys had grown up together and were all very close. I have wonderful memories of the kids putting on plays and skits for the rest of the family to enjoy. They made up tickets and charged us admission to see these one of a kind performances. Then the girls were born with Andrea and then Johnny's first born, Jessica, one year later. John's only son Andrew was born four years after that and the family just continued to grow. We were always in communication with each other. If one of us had a particularly busy week then dad would fill in the gaps. He was more than happy to keep each of his six children up to date on everyone's life. We were raised with the idea that family was everything and always came first. But since our mother died in 1981, those values were held up even higher. We knew what is what like to lose a much loved member of the family. We remembered the fear, the pain and the emptiness. We learned to live without her but we never forgot what it was like to have her and we certainly remembered what it felt like to lose her. We were terrified to go through it all over again.

August 22nd 1994 Josie wrote:

> Appetite is still lousy, no diarrhea today, no nausea, 2 small sores on my bottom lip. Sal came and took Anthony to Dr. L. Everything is okay. I did three loads wash and some dusting. Pretty tired tonight. We also signed a contract with Aquafine water co to install a unit, possibly this week. Good Night.

Chapter 17

A Day in the Life of Josie

August 23rd 1994 Josie wrote:

Still not much appetite and my lip is a little sore, 2 sores. But I took the kids to Harvey's for lunch and then for groceries. They were a big help. Rested when home and then off to Anthony's game. Went for coffee at Joanne and Sergio's and stayed until 11:30 pm. Was so tired to take my Essiac so I went right to sleep.

August 24th 1994 Josie wrote:

I am getting ready to go to Tina's she is having the Restivo clan over. I am picking up Dad on the way. We had a wonderful afternoon. I nibbled on appetizers and had no problem. I had diarrhea once before leaving home and I took my pills. I spoke with Zia Filomena's daughter. Two years ago she had cancer in her throat and had surgery. She is also taking Essiac and swears it makes her feel great. John is not home yet, he had a S.C soccer meeting. It is almost midnight and I think I'll go to sleep.

August 25/94 Josie wrote:

I had a little more energy today and did some dusting and kitchen cleaning. Made tacos for the kids. Paul hated them and Anth and Andrea loved them. One soft movement and a little more appetite. Good Night.

August 26/94 Josie wrote

Busy day, cleaned the house, the installer put in the water filter. My cousins Josie and Mary came with Tony, Josie's son. We had a great time reminiscing. Tina and the kids came too. We had Katie's birthday party tonight. We had a nice evening. No diarrhea or nausea today, ate better also.

Good night.

August 27/94 Josie wrote:

Slept in till 9:45 felt nausea most of the day. Ate a good supper, did 3 loads of wash and later went to the TiCat game and Sal's for coffee. It is 12:10 and I am drinking my tea. Night

August 28/94 Josie wrote:

We didn't make it to church today, the kids slept till 10:30. I made sauce and we had ricotta filled pasta. I had 3 and felt a little nauseated. I had diarrhea a few times earlier in the day and took 2 lomotil pills. We spent most of the day relaxing and doing a jigsaw puzzle. Later at 8:00pm we went to the drive in with lots of junk food. We had a good time. It's late. Goodnight.

August 29/94 Josie wrote:

Today started off very busy once I got up at 10:00 am. I changed my sheets washed and dried, baked some banana breads for Dad and got the kids lunch. Sal came for a visit in time for me to have a nap until it was time for Anth's Dr. L appt. Went to dad's for a short visit and back home for supper and off to soccer. After soccer, Tina etal and Sergio and kids came up to watch Simmer Slam Wrestling. They had a great time. It's 12:05 am now and I'm exhausted. I had diarrhea most of the day. Why?

Goodnight.

August 31/94 Josie wrote:

Up early. Tina is coming at 10:00 am. My appt. with Dr. C is at 10:50 am. He gives me shit because I'm not eating enough. I need more protein and I have to have those BOOST drinks. I have to maintain a level weight throughout chemo sessions he said or I'll die. I told him I'm not going to die and he said I'd be a very miserable person. I have to eat between sessions. My endoscopy he tells me was fine, no irregularities were seen. I lost 2lbs.

Sept. 1 /94 Josie wrote:

Busy day, went to Zellers for school stuff then to Nonno's for a visit and Zia Paola's for tea. A little nausea today after eating about 3 times. Chilly night at Anthony's game. My eyes are very sore and watery and my nose is dripping, maybe allergies have set in. Goodnight.

Sept. 2 /94 Josie wrote:

Today we all went to Pier 4 with Dad, Sal met us there. Dad had a great time thinking about the old days and the old area. We drove by 319 McNab and 26 Wood Street. We had a picnic lunch and sat by the waterfront. I was pretty nauseated today. Why? We went to Cheers for pizza etc. I started to feel pretty sick, got the heaves at home, better later. Tomorrow is a mass for mom at St. Francis at 9:00am. I'll have to get up pretty early.

Goodnight

Sept. 3 /94 Josie wrote:

Up early for a mass at 9:00am for Mom at St. Francis, had coffee at Tina's then took Dad for some groceries. Went home to do lots of laundry. After BBQ supper, we took the kids to see Lion King. We had a great time. I didn't feel nauseated all day.

Sept. 4/94 Josie wrote:

Went to Sunday mass today, the singing was great. Joe and Doris and Dad came to visit, then Rocco and Aurora and Laura came, both visits were very nice. I ate very well today without nausea, If I lay down, I don't feel nauseated. It's almost midnight. I've had my Essiac and going to sleep.

Sept. 5/94 Josie wrote:

Dad organized a BBQ at our place for today. We had a great day and Dad was pretty happy that we were all together. I ate a lot today and had no nausea if I lay down after eating. I've had my tea and ready for the first day of school in the morning. Goodnight.

Chapter 18

Just Another School Year

WHAT IS it about Canadians? We can't wait for the summer months so that we can go on vacation, enjoy the warmer weather and most of all, not have to go to school. But then by August, we somehow start to feel bored, run out of things to do and look through the hundreds of flyers that arrive, advertising all the back to school sales on school supplies. Yes and many of us even start getting tired of the warmer weather and feel like getting into our hoodies and track pants. What about the parents? What a relief to get the kids back to school and out of your hair! How exciting it is to start a new school year, wondering what teacher you will get and who of your friends will be in your class.

I wonder how Josie felt at the start of that year. Did she think that it would be the last time that she would see her children off to start a new year or would this be one of many more to come? Imagine what that is like? Wondering if every pleasure that you enjoy with your children is the last you will ever have. Josie was never burdened by her children and never complained about long summers and wishing that school would start so that she could cart them off. Maybe that is how we should all parent our children, enjoying each experience with them as though it would be our last. I bet if we did that, we would spend more time playing, laughing and listening. Josie did all those things. I truly believe that Josie gave her children a lifetime of lessons and love during her time with them and they are better for having her in their lives.

Sept. 6/94 Josie wrote:

First day of school was hectic; buses were late drove the kids stayed till they were settled. Went back to make sure Andrea got right bus. At Anthony's soccer he strained a ligament. We spent 21/2 hours at St. Joe's ambulatory. We had a very late night. I was so tired.

Sept. 7/94 Josie wrote:

School bus came five minutes late. Andrea and the boys went alone. I was a little hesitant to send Andrea but John assured me she would be fine. The boys took care of her. I had a very relaxing, quiet day once the ironing and laundry was done. Paul lost his game tonight. I felt a little nauseated today but I shouldn't have had chips. I had my Essiac and going to sleep. G-night

Sept. 8/94 Josie wrote:

Better day ate a little more than usual. I think I have a cold, my throat is sore and my nose is dripping and I have a cough. Tonight the cough is bad. The tea calms it down a little but I am really sleepy. Goodnight

Sept. 9 /94 Josie wrote:

I was really busy today dusting, vacuuming and ironing. I rested and watched some videos, made supper and went to Tina's for 7:00pm Weekenders party. Had a great time, in bed by 1:00am.

Sept. 10/94 Josie wrote:

Saturday is a good day to do nothing and that is what I did. I ate pretty well, for supper I had 4 Ricotta shells. I was stuffed. I lay down and it did not feel so bad. John had a golf tourney and didn't get home till 8:00pm not 6:30 as he said. However, we still went for our visit to Frank and Franca's the kids had a whale of a time and the 3 girls had a nice chat alone, we didn't leave till after midnight. I hope Andrea doesn't pick up my cold because she said that her tonsils hurt tonight. We'll have to wait and see. Dad is feeling much better today. His bad cold seems to have worn off. It's almost 1:00am and John is bombed and I'm very tired. I'm drinking my essiac now.

Chapter 19

Three Sisters and a Fair

THIS WAS no ordinary fair. There were no rides or merry go rounds. No cotton candy or silly games that nobody ever wins. No prizes to be won although we had high hopes for the day. The three of us had always arranged the odd outing, but since Josie's illness, we seemed to have wanted to spend more time as a threesome. Going out for a drink was not really our thing. We preferred desserts, movies and good old fortune telling. Yes the psychic fair had come to town and we were not going to miss it. For some reason I am not even sure how we got into all of this. We were born into a very Catholic family. Well for the most part. Dad had his own opinions about the church and the whole lot of..... But mom was a very devout Catholic. Anyways, there was never any talk about the spirit world, just a wonderful place called paradise. I suppose when everything that you know and love is being threatened, you are desperate to look for the answers. I know that we were longing to understand how and why this was happening to Josie and we were searching for someone to tell us that she was going to be okay. So off we go in search and we meet a wonderful lady named Kathy.

Sept. 11/94 Josie wrote:

We went to church today. After lunch Sal and Tina and I went to the Psychic Fair. We met Kathy; she told me I must have more positive thinking to cure myself. I must meditate and think of myself with a glow on all my body parts. She told me that my guardian angel is an old gentleman named Antoine. She also said in previous life, I was a Jewish man who looked down on everyone. I lived in South Africa and Tina's spirit was my wife and she always looked after me and gave me my strength. Another life, I died of hunger and hung on for my life in the water attached by a rope around my back where I have my pain in my back shoulder blades. She suggested that I take parc dàrco (taheebo) and was happy when I told her that I was taking Essiac. She felt my pain in the stomach area and told me I must get rid of my fear and be positive. She said in 1996 she sees me happy and dancing with shivers in my arms and right leg. Also financial security will come next year at this time. Not to worry I must then take a step forward to do what I want to do. My spirit angel Antoine is old because I am not ready to leave this world. He was from dad's side may be an uncle of Dad's. She said Andrea's spirit was an old spirit. I must speak to her as an equal not a child. She is so in tune and sensitive to me but she is not mom's spirit. Kathy will send me and Sal and Tina a relaxation tape to listen at the same time to pass on positive energy. I had my taheebo and essiac tonight. It's 11:30 and I must rest because tomorrow I begin with chemo and radiation. I don't know what to expect. I feel I have to wait and see.

Goodnight.

Chapter 20

Another Round of Chemo

Sept. 12/94 Josie wrote:

First day back from chemo and radiation. It took forever. We had to leave the kids with Joanne till 1:00pm. John took the rest of the day off. I felt nausea as soon as I got home and the heaves 3x. Did feel better later and ate. I'm very tired today, slept a lot today. Goodnight

Sept. 13/94 Josie wrote:

Chemo and radiation day felt much better than yesterday. No nausea and less tired, did nap 1-time, Chiara was over for the pm. Had parent council meeting at 7:00 all was okay. Was in bed early 9:30pm for TV and rest. I'll have my tea at 10:30 pm. Goodnight

Sept. 14/94 Josie wrote:

Chemo and radiation took forever. I saw Dr. B and he said everything was fine. He gave me supplement foods to try out. Was pretty tired but we went to soccer and later in bed early.

Good night.

September 14, 1994 I wrote:

I found out yesterday that me and Chris are going to be parents.

Sept. 15, 1994 I wrote:

I am in the sun room with a cup of hot water, lemon and honey. Supposedly I need to limit my caffeine intake now. I am at home and I have had bronchitis since Sunday. It is now Thursday. So much has happened this past week.

Last week was a very difficult week for me. I was very tired, pale and stressed out because of work. I get very worked up about things and I suppose that needs to change too. I thought I was getting my period but I never did and I kept having this craving for veal cutlets. I don't usually crave things and if I do it passes. By Saturday, it still didn't pass and I told Chris that we needed to get some veal cutlets at the local grocery store. He agreed but said he had a surprise for me first. I do like surprises. He took me to the psychic fair in Burlington. I was very excited and met a woman there who told me that my spirit angel was named Lilla. Seems like a nice Italian name. According to the woman, Lilla told me to go with my dream, my career dream and not to be afraid. I would be very successful. Go with your big plan she kept saying. She also told me to forgive my father and that this was very important. Maybe she saw that dad was going to die and I needed to forgive him. I didn't ask and I don't think she would have told me anyways. She said that dad didn't mean to do those things to me. She picked up that I resented him for holding me back. She said that he is narrow minded and that is all he knew. I really tried to be reasonable with dad. He won't listen to me or take me seriously. I hope I don't make those same mistakes with my kids someday. She suggested that I needed to forgive dad and to do that I needed to write out my feelings on paper, read it seven times and then burn it.

She sensed my anxieties, my difficulty in breathing, nervous stomach and pain in my back. She attributed all of this to a past life. She told me that Chris and I were together in a past life and that he fell off a cliff and broke his neck – seems to explain why he is afraid of cleaning the eaves troughs. It was quite a day and I was not sure what to make of all this new information. I was tired but I still wanted those veal cutlets.

The next day, I woke up with a sore throat but I went back to the psychic fair with my sisters. A lady named Kathy felt that Josie was going to be fine and she needed to be more positive and face her fear. Easier said than done! By Monday, I was even sicker and still no period so I made an appointment. As it turned out, I had bronchitis and a sinus infection. I took a blood test while I was there which came back positive by the next day. I am pregnant and contrary to the doctor's recommendation to keep it a secret until the three months has passed, I was right on the phone to Josie and shared with her the good news. She was very happy for us and offered her congratulations, but I know what she was thinking. We were both thinking the same thing. I called Tina and told her the news and it was a strange conversation too because we were all thinking the same thing. Surprisingly it was very comforting to tell dad and for once I didn't wish it was mom. I'm glad it was dad. I could tell that he was really happy. I think he was starting to wonder what else was wrong with his youngest daughter for at thirty-two years old, she still had no kids. In the next few days we told the rest of my siblings and some of our friends. It still doesn't seem real. I am terrified to be a mother, afraid that I won't be much good at it. I feel happy and sad all at the same time. It is amazing how this life will grow inside me for nine months. It is truly a miracle.

Chapter 21

More of Josie's Daily Entries

Sept. 15/94 Josie wrote:

Today was just radiation it was over within 20 minutes. I went to dad's directly because we were going to the ambulatory hospital to check Dad's chest, that took over two hours. But he got thoroughly checked and antibiotics. Came home exhausted but I called Mary C for brewing recipe. I'll make it on Sunday. I rested all evening, no nausea today just queezie and tired.

Goodnight.

Sept. 16/94 Josie wrote:

Busy morning after a 9:00am nap I vacuumed and did 2 loads and dusted. Radiation appt was 2:45 pm so Chiara came at 2:15 for the kids. I was back in time however, Chiara did my veal cutlets then we had chiropractor at 4:30 stopped at Big V for supplies and home to cook supper. John came home very late and we left for Nancy's at 8:00pm. Michael (baby) 2nd birthday was fun. He is sooo cute. It's 11:00pm

Goodnight.

Sept. 17/94 Josie wrote:

Its 11:30 pm I'm totally wiped. Today was an 8:00 am start with S.C soccer tournament. Anthony lost the cup game, Paul won his consolation and he also played against a rep team and won. Then Paul played with Wally in another rep game and they lost. After all that we were at Tina's for the rest of the evening. When we got to Tina's, her neighbor approached us about buying their house. They want to move next May or June and won't use a real estate company if we are really interested. It's too complicated. I can't think about that right now.

Goodnight

Sept. 18/94 Josie wrote:

Went to church a little hectic. I was almost too tired to go but I did. I have my period and feel cramps and have some clotting and good flow. I spent most of the day resting and watching T.V. I ate cereal with milk, pasta w/sauce and ½ a meatball, later some peanut butter and nutella with melba toast. Then I had some cookies ½ tangerine then my essiac. Goodnight 1st day of period.

Sept. 19/94 Josie wrote:

Sal came over this morning and we went to radiation together. After that we went bra shopping then home. Dad had an appt with Dr. R and I with Dr. Z. I gave him my forms for CPP disability and he gave me a B12 shot. I was very very tired today after supper I rested and prepared the rest of my Essiac batch. It's bottled and ready.

Sept. 20/94 Josie wrote:

Late appt today after groceries came home. Chiara came and I rested. Bit of nausea no diarrhea. Goodnight.

Sept. 21/94 Josie wrote:

My appt was early. They want to take more x-rays tomorrow on my kidneys. Sarah and Tina and Sal came after lunch for a visit. I felt pretty tired after supper though. We went to open house at the school. It went well. The kids all have great teachers. I was really tired by 11:00 went to bed.

Sept. 22/94 Josie wrote:

Today is busy. I have a 10:15 after that I went shopping for a pair of pants and a vest. Came home for lunch and back to the hospital for x-rays of my kidneys. They decided to prepare a block during radiation so as not to damage the kidneys, It went quickly I was back by 3:15 even though Chiara came up to meet the kids. I drove her home. I ate well tonight but tomorrow is a busy one so I must rest.

Sept. 23/94 Josie wrote:

My appt was 8:30 I had blood work done. Made it right on 9:30 for the bus to the Ancaster Fair. We had a great day but by 3:00pm I was spent. Rested all day. Sergio came to start the painting/scrapping/priming. Rest all evening and in bed by 11:00pm. I felt nausea quite a bit today but no diarrhea. Goodnight for now.

Sept. 24/94 Josie wrote:

Sergio came at 8:00 am but no go because it rained, so they went to Alex's place for pepper bbq. I rested for most of the day except for ironing. Tonight we went to Copps with Alex and Marney for the Elvis Tour Skating Show. It was fantastic. We went to their place for coffee afterwards and home at 1:00 am

Sept. 25/94 Josie wrote:

We made it to church this morning. John played his last soccer game. We spent the rest of the pm at Chiara and Mario's for lunch. It was too late to visit Dad. We came home at 9:00 and I passed out asleep by 10:00.

Sept. 26/94 Josie wrote:

Andrea was home sick today. It seems like a cold and runny nose. Sal came and Tina came also for lunch. Sal made some soup for me. I was busy this am doing laundry and bathroom jobs. My appt. was at 3:15 Sal stayed for the kids Andrea napped for 2 hours today. They took x-rays again. I am very drowsy tonight. I had my essiac.

Sept. 27/94 Josie wrote:

Met with the dietician Karen today. She gave me some samples, nothing interesting. Then had radiation. It was fine then went to see Dr. C. He said we would wait for another endoscopy and gave me a new prescription for nausea. Had parent council meeting and it went fine. After we had coffee at Tim's with Angela, Sue and Deb.

Sept. 28/94 Josie wrote:

Early appt at 9:00 saw Dr. B everything looks fine. He gave me a new med for the dumping /nausea.

Did lunch duty came home to rest and went out for Festitalia dinner. I ate okay just slight nausea. Very tired went to bed late.

Sept. 29/94 Josie wrote:

Brought all my meds so Wayne could see what I should take. I feel much clearer on that he stopped everything except the lomotil (diarrhea) Stemtil for nausea only when bad. And the new med, Dr. B prescribed as a steroid. It increases appetite and slows digestion to prevent dumping. Boys had optometrist appt and it went well. Anthony re-adjusted and Paul just a check till next year. Boys had cartooning at 5:30 pm -7:00pm they love it. They had showers and all are ready for bed. I stayed up until 11:00 and slept on the couch. John woke me at 12:00

Sept. 30/94 Josie wrote:

I spent the whole day at home. I did laundry, vacuuming and dusting. I ate very well today. The new medication from Dr. B seems to work very well. I don't feel nauseated . Just a slight quickening of my heart and vibrating in my bowels. It's 11:30. I am going to bed now.

Oct. 1/94 Josie wrote:

Easy Saturday morning, loafed around ate but felt a little nausea today after each meal. Andrea had 1st day at Baby Jazz w/Nicole only 4 little ones in the class. I think she'll love it. The boys convinced John and I to go to Eaton's warehouse and we purchased a 13" T.V for them and a HIFI stereo VCR Panasonic both, on a deferred payment plan till April /95. We had a pizza supper and watched T.V till late.

Oct. 2/94 Josie wrote:

Up for church at 11:30 after mass we went to Tina's for a nice day and supper. Felt very tired today slept at Tina's. Ate very well not so much nausea. Stayed up until 11:30 pm.

Oct. 3/94 Josie wrote:

Early appt 9:00 rushed off the kids. Treatment was pretty quick told them about my side pain. Went to Sears after then home met Tina at Eastgate for a shopping Spree. Home for the kids supper, clean up, showers and bed. Goodnight world!

Oct. 4/94 Josie wrote:

Early morning again . I saw the dietician after radiation and have lost no weight this week. I ate very well today only once nausea. I've been very tired today. Chiara came did ironing for me. I rested most of the night. In bed by 11:00 pm Goodnight.

Oct. 5/94 Josie wrote:

9:30 am today saw Wayne and Dr. R who is filling in for Dr. B. Told him about side pain wasn't concerned could be a pulled muscle. Did lunch duty today, and stayed for info on Hepatitis B injections for Anthony. Went to Eaton's warehouse to pick up VCR and T.V. Kids are thrilled and Chris came to hook up everything. Sal came later and we went for a haircut at Annette's new house. I seem to have extra energy tonight. It's 11:20 pm and I'm still awake.

Oct. 7/94 Josie wrote:

Today was blood work and treatment which finished by10:00 and went to school for 10:30. Thanksgiving celebration for Paul. I came home and slept for an hour and went to Dad's for fruit and tomatoes. Later came home and rested most of the evening I slept and slept and slept.

Oct 8/94 Josie wrote:

Up early 7:30 am. Sergio was here at 8:00 we had coffee and they started working outside. Andrea and I went shopping then to dance. The boys hung around home today. Dad and Tina came over tonight for a visit. We'll see each other tomorrow at Sal's for Thanksgiving dinner.

Oct. 9/94 Josie wrote:

We made church and then went to Sal and Chris' for a wonderful Thanksgiving supper. Joe and family came, Tina and Rock, dad and us. We had a wonderful time. I felt good after eating. The desert made me a little nauseated.

Then I was fine. In bed at 11:30. I feel very tired.

Oct. 10/94 Josie wrote:

Spent a lazy morning this holiday Thanksgiving Monday. Made some quick lasagna today. Kids ate almost the whole two trays. Went later in the pm for a nature walk at King's Forest. Mr. DM lost his keys in the woods and had to go find them while Andrea and I froze out by the car. Luckily Paul found them then we went to Claudio and Nancy's to give Patrick his movie passes for his birthday. We were home by 8:00pm. Andrea had a bath and we just relaxed the evening. Tomorrow is another treatment day. I'd better get some sleep. I got a busy one.

Oct. 11/94 Josie wrote:

Treatment was quick today. I saw dietician lost no weight still 46.6. Home by 10:00 am went to school mass and Sal came by with leftovers. Listened to Kathy's tape today it was great. After supper went to Chiara's. Ugo and Yolanda are here from Australia.

Oct. 12/94 Josie wrote:

Had to wait today saw Dr. B everything fine. He is not concerned about the pain in left side. Weight still okay, no loss. Went to Franca's to learn that Anthony got hurt at school. Went to school Anthony seems to have a concussion. Brought him to St. Joe's Ambulatory diagnosed as a concussion, no other affects, x-rays okay. Home at 4:00pm. Anthony was hungry and rest all evening. So did I (exhausted)

Oct. 13/94 Josie wrote:

Left for school early to get Anthony's hepatitis B shot but they suggested it be postponed for now because of his trauma from the concussion. Mario stayed at home with Anthony till I came back from the hospital all went well, back pretty quick rested today did laundry and ironing, cooked supper. Brought the kids to art class and relaxed most of the evening. It seems that I have only 3 more days of radiation. We'll see?

Oct. 14/94 Josie wrote:

Therapy was very quick had blood tests done. Only 2 days left. After went to Sears shopped and then for groceries after I went to school and found Anthony sick waiting for me. I brought him right to Dr. Z he said it was normal to still be dizzy and went to Dad's. He gave me fruit and $100.00. Came home made sauce. We crashed most of the night on T.V. Had a bad bout of diarrhea. Feel better now very tired. John's at HSR stag. Home at 12:30am.

Oct. 15/94 Josie wrote:

I got up early today and I don't know why. Made pancakes for the kids went to the mall for Andrea's gifts. John went out with the boys. Sal and Chris came over and Tina and boys for a roast beef supper. Then we went to Brantford to see Melodie. What an interesting woman.

She gave us tons of information and some herb combinations for all three of us. She pinpointed various things to strengthen the immune system and she swears by the tea of life (essiac). Told me to add two more ounces a day along with another herb which we purchased tonight. We are going to try for a month's supply and see her again. I have had my tea. GN

Chapter 22

No One is Listening!!

To HAVE chemotherapy or not to have chemotherapy? That is the question. Damned if you do and damned if you don't. I remember Josie and me talking about her decision to go ahead with chemo. For the record, it was not something that she wanted to do. We all know at least in those days, that getting chemo made you feel worse before you would ever feel better. Josie was advised of the side effects; nausea, cold sores, fatigue and let's not forget, hair loss. In spite of all these side effects, there were no guarantees that her life would be saved. All this information did not stack up in favor of chemo, but the reality was, what if you don't take the chemo? Then what? Would you be wondering if the chemo would have saved your life? So after all the debate Josie decided that she would have to go ahead with it and hoped that it would have all been worth it. Well after several treatments of chemo and a few rounds of radiation which seemed the lesser of the two evils, Josie called it quits. What a courageous woman!

Oct. 17/94 Josie wrote:

> Today Dad's test went fine. They found one
> polyp and took it out. On the other hand, my

radiation is almost over and I see Dr. F today. He tries to talk me out of quitting my treatments but I am very sure that I don't want anymore. He disagrees. I'm confused and tried but I am not sure that a few more treatments can guarantee me anything. It's in God's hands now. I'll do everything possible without making myself sick with chemo. John and I both agree on this decision. Tonight I feel scared. I am so vulnerable that it scares me. After radiation I saw Karen (dietician) I lost only .6kg then waited forever for Dr. B. He's pleased with my progress and recommends an endoscopy later on in January because there is too much inflammation at this point. I'll discuss that with Dr. C on Tuesday's appt. I'm to see Dr. B in December and after that I saw Barb to tell her no more chemo. So I'm booked Nov 14 to see Dr. F she says. I can discuss further chemo with him. They don't get it, they're not listening!

My very first book, On Death and Dying was by the infamous, Elisabeth Kubler-Ross.1 It was recommended and given to me by my religion teacher at my high school during the time when my own mother was dying. As I hold this small paperback book in my hand now, I can see that it was well used and referenced. It was given to me in 1980 and with its pages coming apart at the seams; it brings me back to that young, innocent girl who was terrified to be left behind. This book became my bible and gave me the strength to make sense of the situation around me that made no sense to me at all.

[1]Elisabeth Kubler-Ross, On death and dying: (New York; Macmillan Publishing CO.,INC 1969)

It has been so many years since I have read each word on these pages but I still remember the stages of dying. The first stage was denial and the shock of receiving such sad and devastating news. The second stage was anger. Naturally feeling like why me and what did I do to deserve this would result in becoming angry at others and God. Thirdly, the bargaining stage is the negotiation for a little more time. Depression becomes the fourth stage when you realize that bargaining for more time may not work and then somehow you eventually come into the final stage of Acceptance. However, acceptance of what, that your life is coming to an end? Or an acceptance in a spiritual sense where you must embrace your circumstances. I am thinking now as I did then of all the stages that we all went through. This book was like an instruction manual and always let me know what we could expect next. It gave me knowledge and with that knowledge I was able to prepare myself and in turn my loved ones for what was to come. I remember one of the overall themes in this book was for terminally ill patients to die with dignity. I remember being very supportive of this thought and did what I could to give my mother the respect that she needed to die with dignity. I often wonder if I or the medical community gave Josie that same respect throughout her battle with this disease. Did she feel heard and understood? Or were we all stuck in denial?

Oct. 20/94 Josie wrote:

> Left at 10:00 dad got his flu shot we went to the Bank and groceries. We had lunch together and a nap. Dad insisted on giving me $500 to be able to buy the herbals from Melody. I am very grateful. Tonight Andrea and I went to Char's for Just Kids party. I got her some nice things. It's almost midnight. Goodnight.

Oct. 21/94 Josie wrote:

PA day today Tina's boys came. They were all pretty good. Anthony's one brace piece dislodged. Matty hit him with a stuffed animal. I made a batch of Essiac today, vacuumed and dusted. The dishwasher got repaired $81.00. Tina came and Anthony and I went for his Hepatitis B shot. Sal and Chris came with ultrasound pictures the baby is tiny. Chiara and Mario came for coffee. It's late. 12:16 Good night

Oct. 22/94 Josie wrote:

Slow Saturday not much going this morning. John went for wine with Dad at noon and after dance, Andrea and I cleaned her room right out. All the baby stuff is gone to Sal and Chris and all the clothes to Charlene. Tonight we went to a movie with Sal and Chris and Tina and Rock. Love Affair; a little slow on the action still a tear jerker. We came to our place for tea and coffee and pastries later.

October 23, 1994 I wrote:

What a lazy weekend it has been for both of us. The pregnancy has been going well so far. We had an ultrasound and all is well. I saw the baby for the first time. I heard the heart beating quickly and felt some fluttering but still too small to look like a baby. My due date is May 18th and I am 10 weeks and 4 days. Chris of course was there and he was totally ecstatic. He is positive it is a girl, but I always pictured myself having a boy first. The thought of having a daughter is a thrill. I hope that I will be a good role model for a daughter. Josie and Andrea have been so generous. They went through all the toys this weekend and we brought home boxes of stuff last night. The three sisters and our hubbies went to the movies to see Love Affair. We had a great time. I feel at peace. I feel very calm. Chris has even noticed. I want my baby to be born healthy. I want to do what comes natural. I will have my two sisters to help me and offer me guidance. Josie is going to be around for the long haul. She decided to discontinue the chemo and I support her decision. She is now 100lbs. She needs to build up weight. Her face looks great. She is so beautiful. I know she will be well. There is no way that she will be taken from us. She has been taking the essiac and a bunch of other herbs. We have opened our minds to completely new things and this is good for us. We are keeping a positive outlook. I love my sisters, both of them and I refuse to let either of them go.

Chapter 23

It's Business as Usual

Oct. 23/94 Josie wrote:

Busy Monday tidied the house and picked up pizza money dropped off choc money and counted. Went to Joanne's after supper for Weekenders party with Chiara and Tina,home by 11:00. Goodnight tomorrow is my appt. with Dr. C.

Oct. 25/94 Josie wrote:

Saw Dr. C at 9:00am with John, all is well. He was not upset that I'm stopping chemo. We discussed the dumping he said it might never go away. Maybe lessen, I'd get used to it. Had breakfast with Dad went to school then home to count pizza money. Brought Paul to Grimsby for soccer after MacDonald s and home.

Oct. 28/94 Josie wrote:

Drove to Roller Gardens today. Kids had a ball. Left for awhile to Sears to buy a new coat on sale. Met John downtown to bring papers for disability ate some nuts and felt pretty nauseated. Saw Dr. W, the chiropractor, he agrees with my decision to stop chemo and he advises to up my vitamin C. After supper John went to Johnny's to cook tripe. We watched TV and went to bed by 11:00.

Oct. 29/94 Josie wrote:

The day looks good and we're going to the pumpkin patch. We met Tina and Roc at Franca and Frank's and left for Brantford where we met Sal and Chris. We had a great time. It was a little cool and windy. We were home by 4:00pm. I started and finished 4 loads of wash, made supper and Andrea's cake is baked. We'll decorate tomorrow. Clocks go back for an hour so we can sleep in a bit. It's going to be a busy day for Andrea's party.

Oct. 30/94 Josie wrote:

Off to church with the usual rush. Back to clean house and decorate cake for Andrea's party. Everyone came and we had a great time. She got a lot of beautiful things, clothes and toys. Everyone left by 10:00pm. I felt a little sick after I had some cake. I went to bed at midnight.

Oct. 31/94 Josie wrote:

Halloween six years ago today, I went into labor w/Andrea. She was a happy Snow White. Not too many kids. I'm really surprised maybe 40.

Nov. 1/94 Josie wrote:

Andrea is happy today. They will announce her name and birthday on the P.A. Paul played soccer, it poured rain all day. We treated the kids to Mac Donald's after soccer.

Nov. 3/94 Josie wrote:

Last few days I have been too sleepy at night to write. I baked several dozen choc chips tonight. Anthony needs them for raffle tomorrow.

Nov. 4/94 Josie wrote:

Went for lunch duty today. I enjoyed seeing all the kids. Went to dads for lunch. Tina and Sal came too. I was to nauseated to eat. It seems like everything I eat this week no matter how small makes me feel sick, the dumping effect is very bad. Maybe it will pass? Just rested and watched T.V tonight.

Nov. 5/94 Josie wrote:

Slept in till 9:00 am felt pretty good. Still nause-ated after eating most of the day. Did 4 loads of wash and some ironing. Had a bubble bath w/ Andrea, in bed at 11:30.

Chapter 24

Just Another Lazy Sunday

Nov. 6 1994 I wrote:

Need to rest. It's Sunday today. I woke up at 7:30 am and had tons of energy. So I made a pot of sauce and chicken soup. We have been cleaning and doing laundry. Yesterday we bought a video camera for when the baby comes. I am so exhausted now. I am in the sun room and it is very comfortable. I haven't spoken with Josie today. She has the bazaar after church. I get so worried about her. I have an ache, a feeling of uncertainty. I want things to be the way they were. This kind of worry is too painful. On most days I feel she will be okay and then on others days I think, oh my God how is this going to end? I love her so much.

Nov. 6/94 Josie wrote:

Church today found out Fr. Jim's mother had a heart attack. After mass we attended the church bazaar and the kids didn't win anything. We had left overs for lunch and off to Christina's semi final B-Ball then to dad's for a while and back for game 2 of the finals. They lost.

Nov. 7/94 Josie wrote:

Car (Corsica) got towed away today after failed attempts to get it started. Will be ready in the am. Sal took Anthony and I for his pre-op appt. at St. Joe's. It took a few hours and back by 3:00pm. Bob to show John how to change the filter.

Nov. 8/94 Josie wrote:

Went with John downtown to pick up the car. $325.00 later. Came home and did some wash and ironing. Went for interview for Andrea. All's well. Off to soccer for Paul and Paesano's for pizza with Paul and Rita. Back a little late at 9:50pm in bed for midnight.

Nov. 9/94 Josie wrote:

Stayed home this morning did some laundry and ironing. Took Anthony to see Dr. H at 1:00pm. She checked Anthony and described some surgery and side effects (bruising). John's AGM for SC soccer. He was nominated and elected president. The problems are just beginning for him.

Nov. 10/94 Josie wrote:

Talked to Kathy about parent council stuff. Went for groceries and then to Dad's. Spent a few hours with dad and we had lunch. Went to Sears for some shopping for some clothes for me and Andrea. John went to play soccer and I rested and watched T.V

Nov. 11/94 Josie wrote:

I'm writing catch up for a few days.

Nov. 12/94 Josie wrote:

We slept in and brought kids to Sal's office for the Star Trek mini convention. It was pretty good and then off to Sal and Chris' for some supper. Dad came over too.

Nov. 13/94 Josie wrote:

Up early to see the Miracle on 34th street at the Centre. Movie was great then off to Harvey's for lunch. Back home to do laundry and ironing. John was busy running the bingo.

Nov. 14/94 Josie wrote:

Appt 9:00am at the cancer hospital had blood work done. I saw Dr. F he doesn't press the matter and wants to see me in February after all my tests. We had a mini parent council meeting at Pam and Mike's to discuss guidelines.

Chapter 25

Never a Dull Moment

On Nov. 15/94 Josie wrote:

Anthony gets ready this morning for his surgery. We arrive at 10:00 am kill some time til 11:30 am. Anthony is pretty hungry by noon. The nurse has trouble with his IV, can't find a vein. We waited until 12:30pm. Dr. H comes to get him and John and I wait for surgery to end at 1:00pm. Dr. H came out and told us all went well and we could see him soon. Within 5 minutes I was in recovery with him. He felt confused and had a throbbing eye. They gave him tylenol in the IV. He was very good. At 2:00pm we were in the room and he slept for a few hours. We were home by 4:00pm. Chiara was home with the kids. Tina brought soup. Paul played soccer all was quiet at 9:00pm and I passed out. Anthony slept all night well.

Nov. 16/94 Josie wrote:

Anthony had a little crusty on his eye and it is pretty red. We had post -op appt. for 1:30pm. All is well and eye appears straighter. We will know better in six weeks time. John had exec meeting for soccer at our house tonight.

Nov. 22/94 Josie wrote:

Many days have passed and Anthony's eye is doing fine. He went to school yesterday. This past weekend, Sergio and John painted the house. It looks fabulous. They started prepping on Friday and painted all day Saturday. I stayed at Dad's on Friday night and all Saturday. Came home at Saturday night at 9:00pm everything was tidied and clean. Sal came over today and we put some things on the walls. I still need a few new things?? After Paul's game, we went to Chiaras, her surgery is Thursday. Tomorrow, Tina and I go to Dr. L.

Nov. 25/94 Josie wrote:

A few days missed but nothing to report. Tina and I went to Dr. L on Wednesday. Her cervix is fallen not much can be done until it affects her cycle and urinating. We went to Eastgate after for a Chinese lunch. I ate so much and hardly felt sick. We did some shopping for Christmas. Thursday was sub day, it was pretty hectic but all went well w/o too many problems. Today was a PA day the kids were pretty good. I left them for half an hour for the interviews at the school and the house was still standing.

Tonight we went to Mississauga to see Marcie and pray the Rosary. Marcie was told of my illness and anointed me with holy oil and told me to take more with me to anoint myself each day. I cried again tonight. I couldn't help it. Kay wants us to come to the Fatima Shrine on Dec

17 by bus, I look forward to it. Thank God for happiness and family.

Dec. 23/94 Josie wrote:

A month has passed, I have been falling asleep on the sofa after my tea and it's too hard to write every night. I should take the time each morning to record my thoughts. Anyways, I've been feeling pretty good. I saw Dr. B Dec 12, he said everything was fine. What he can tell by poking around on the outside beats me? The last few days I've been feeling very gurgly in my bowel area. It scares me so much I remember that feeling now I know what it is in my stomach. Needless to say, this has been a sad week. I feel like crying all the time. I'll have to wait for Dr. C's tests in January to be done. It's almost Christmas we'll be at Tina's on the 24th and Sal's on the 25th. Tonight we exchanged gifts at Chiara's. We had a good time. Tomorrow I must start early to prepare the lasagna and make a desert for Christmas day. I'll settle down and write more often after the holiday is over. Goodnight.

Chapter 26

Merry Christmas and Happy New Year

Dec. 24/94 Josie wrote:

Christmas Eve. A busy day making lasagna and cheesecake. We went to Tina and Rocks for dinner. We had a wonderful time. All the kids were happy and the adults too. It was a very late night. Tomorrow it's off to Sal and Chris' for more food!

Merry Christmas

Christmas is really my favorite holiday of all time. It is the celebration of the birth of Christ. Happy Birthday Jesus! But I have to admit that I love the lights, the glitter and all the bling, not to mention the hustle and the bustle of the shopping and yes the food. It seems as though this is one time of the year that we can indulge and not feel bad about it. I don't just mean food, I also mean spending money. We often find ourselves spending way beyond our means to get that perfect gift regardless of the cost. Sure it is a stressful time for many but it all leads to that magical celebration.

Thank God mom insisted that we take all those super 8 movies to capture all those precious memories of when we were kids. I think mom loved Christmas too. It was a time when she brought out all her best stuff and showcased her cooking talents. From what I can remember, dad was always by her side in the kitchen too. Together they made sure that Christmas was a special time for us all. As the family grew larger, we spent bits and pieces of it together. Mom expected that. Even after she died we still managed to share a meal but it was difficult and it became too stressful for dad despite everyone's help. So we moved the celebration over to my sisters Tina's house and for many years enjoyed wonderful Christmases. Christmas 1994 would be no exception. We enjoyed and indulged and we exchanged hugs, kisses and gifts. We laughed and joked but there was a quiet uneasiness and I know that we all felt it. None of us wanted to give into it but it was an unspoken fear that this Christmas as we knew it, would be our last. What a year it had been for Josie and for all of us. She was so strong and courageous. That Christmas, Josie showcased her cooking talents and made the best lasagna and cheesecake that we had ever eaten. As we welcomed the New Year, we remained hopeful that our family would be blessed with the miracle of life for our new baby and for Josie.

January 8/95 Josie writes:

> Christmas went well and it's almost back to reality. In the morning, I have to prepare three tired kids for school and get to Dr. C's by 10:00am. I can do it! I don't know what to tell him except that I have been eating constantly and feeling very little nausea from the dumping. But--- I'm scared because I feel that same rumbling in my abdomen area. It could just be

my new mechanics working away at my food, or it could be the worst possible thing and the cancer is growing again. I have to write it down. I know I have to think positive but God in heaven, how strong can I be without fearing this damned disease. Nobody will talk about it with me, because they're more scared than I am. I know I have to wait for all the tests to be done. But deep in my heart I'm afraid and I can't get the fear out of my head. I'm praying and I want to believe the best but I'm still so scared.

And there it is. After reading about a thousand loads of laundry and hundreds of trips to dads and multiple meetings at the school for parent council, we finally hear the truth about what Josie was feeling.

Chapter 27

Sunday Visits

THERE IS so much talk around the complexity of the mother daughter relationship, but very little about the relationship between a father and a daughter. Growing up, my father was not the easiest person to talk to and my sisters and I often feared him. When we were young, I remember Sunday afternoons were often reserved for visiting. There was a process and it went something like this. My sisters and I would be just waking up to the smell of homemade chicken soup because that is what we always had on Sundays. I would hear my mother suggesting to my father that it might be nice to do some visiting. He would ask her who she had in mind and then my mother would tell him. Sometimes I got the feeling by her tone that she too was afraid to ask him. At times an argument would break out and at other times my dad was agreeable. He was often very unpredictable. My mother then would take it from there and make the necessary calls that would complete the arrangements. Sometimes my sisters and I were not keen on going depending who it was. But despite the fact that my sisters were old enough, staying at home alone was never an option. So we would get ourselves ready, usually in our Sunday best and haul ourselves into a taxi. My dad did not drive, nor did my mother. In those days, nobody's mother drove. I was always a little embarrassed that we did not have a car and had to take a taxi or public transportation. Dad would often say he was an alphabeto which meant he was illiterate. But back then there were a lot of immigrants that couldn't read or write and they were driving around the city. Anyways it's something we got used to.

I usually had a good time at these visits especially if there were kids there my age. It was often a nice way to spend a Sunday afternoon. It was nice to see my parents interacting with people their own age. We would often have a light snack, food and drink. But my dad always had a watchful eye. He would from a distance monitor how many chips we took from the bowl. If he felt that we had taken one too many chips, then he would widen his big blue eyes and stare at us. He never had to say a word, we just knew that this was the "You took too many chips" look. But I guess in those days, dads were the disciplinarians. He worked and mom stayed home to raise us kids and manage the house. Dad never laid a hand on us girls. He did his fair share of yelling and giving us that cold stare, but he never hit us. As for the boys, those were different times and most kids were threatened with the belt in those days.

My father was always an excellent provider and we never went without, as my mother used to say. My mother handled everything else that went on in the house. So I suppose when she became ill, my dad who had just retired from his thirty years at the steel foundry, had to take on a lot more of the responsibilities. Not to mention caring for a terminally ill wife. I never really stopped to think how that must have been for my father back then. Grieving can be such a selfish act. We often only see our own pain and miss what others around us are going through. We were all feeling the pain but we still had work, school and our own young families. Even my sisters were in the midst of planning their wedding.

Dad was home with mom, day in and day out. I am sure it was an adjustment for them both. Up until then, mom had had the whole house to herself. Having to share it with dad I am sure was a difficult transition especially since she was vulnerable and needed him to care for her. My parents had been together for over forty years , many of those years were spent having children and raising them, making the sacrifices my parents reminded us of so many times. My father worked and made money while my mother stayed at home, economizing by baking bread, cookies and always preparing home cooked meals. There was no such thing as eating out in our family. I'm not even sure anyone in our circle even ate out. Because we didn't, we just assumed no one else did either. So you figure, all those hard years of having kids and making sacrifices and then you get cancer. Mom had just turned fifty eight years old when they discovered the cancer in her women parts. Dad was sixty four when he retired and started taking care of mom. Mom went for a round of chemotherapy and decided that it wasn't for her. The rest of her years were spent at home with the gentle care of our very own Dr. R who came to our house on the way home to his. Our parents were very grateful for his excellent care and compassionate bedside manner. To show their appreciation, there were always a few gallons of wine put aside for the holidays for the good doctor and his family to enjoy. My dad was a generous and thoughtful man.

Over the five years since her diagnosis, mom's health deteriorated. She had become very thin and frail. No longer was she the full figured, energetic mother who was bustling about in the kitchen. The disease had taken more of my mother than her good looks. It took away her spirit and robbed her of the joy that she was entitled to in her later years. I know that there was an anger in her, a resentment within her that was deep and she often begrudged those that enjoyed good health and a zest for living. As a result, she came across as a bitter woman and although it wasn't pretty, you could understand where she was coming from. My mother did not want to die but she wanted to be rid of the pain and put an end to the quality of life that had become her reality.

Mom had had a lot of time to reflect upon her life. I remember all too well our private conversations usually on a Sunday, when everyone was out. I would stay home with mom because she was not able to be left alone. It was our time to visit and mom's time to talk about her feelings, her illness and her pending death. I was only eighteen at the time but I knew that this time that I was spending with my mother would be time that I would treasure for the rest of my life. I am so grateful. I remember just blurting it out one day and asking my mother if she was afraid to die. She seemed stunned, but yet relieved that finally the door had been opened and she was given the opportunity to express her feelings. She told me that she was not afraid to die. She was waiting to be taken into the arms of God but she did not want to leave her family, her children and the life that she knew. She especially did not want to leave me. She felt I was too young to be without a mother and was concerned about leaving me with my dad. Mom was always the buffer between us. I knew I could always find comfort with my mother. Now that she was leaving, who would provide that comfort for me now? I remember telling my mother that I did not want her to die. I couldn't imagine what her life was like. I no longer wanted her to suffer with this disease and told her that when it was time for her to go, that I would be okay. I really didn't know where these words were coming from. I was eighteen years old and far too young to be left without a mother. I didn't want my mother to die and leave me with dad yet I wasn't so sure that I was going to be okay. But somehow I felt I was guided and knew that my frail little mom needed to hear those words from me. My mother told me that she appreciated these private visits, and often looked forward to everyone being out so that we could sit together and talk.

Mom always referred to me as her Savior. In fact, that is the meaning of my name. I never really understood what that meant until that moment. She told me she had known that she was dying despite my dad's wish to keep it from her. After all these years, I still don't understand why he made this decision to keep my mother's illness from her, and why we were not to discuss it. I learned many valuable lessons about life and about myself. I learned how important it is for all people to be heard especially the sick and the dying. My mother had lived a life where she was devoted to her family and to her children. All that she did, she did for us and she deserved the opportunity to reflect and express her feelings about her life and about her death.

I am still so grateful that I was given the courage and the insight to know that this is what she needed. I am a better person for having that experience in my life. You know when they say you learn the most from tragedy and sadness and you go ya ya ya. This is one of those examples. Through this deeply painful and personal experience, I also learned that I had a gift and that I had shared that gift with my mother. That experience has set the path that I would take in my life and in my career as a listener and a helper. I suppose these days cancer is a household name. Everyone knows at least one person who has cancer or has been touched by the deadly disease. But back in the late 70's it was not as widely talked about. It was a taboo topic and I think that many even thought cancer was contagious. As ridiculous as that sounds now, it's just the way it was; in my family anyways.

Chapter 28

The Gift

MY MOTHER died on Friday September 4, 1981 at 7:00pm. In fact it was the start of the long weekend; the one that marks the end of the summer and the beginning of another school year. Mom was very excited as she was expecting her niece and husband from Italy who she had not seen since she left Italy almost thirty years ago. They were planning to stay at our house and I was helping my mother prepare. She had asked me to clear out a few dresser drawers in her bedroom for them to store their belongings. I found it odd as we were not expecting them for several months. I could never say no to mom and did what she asked.

That particular year I was beginning a new chapter in my life. I had big dreams to live away from home and that summer I applied to several universities outside of the city. I was accepted but decided that given my mother's pending death, I should stay close to home. And I did, but she died at the start of "frosh week." That is the week when all the new students participate in lots of activities, festivities and drink a lot of booze. Naturally, I did not attend. I had my place and that was with my mother.

There are many ways a person can die. My mother lived with cancer for five years and then within a week, her life had all come to an end. I remember the weekend before she died, I and a few friends organized a beach day as our last hoorah before we all went our separate ways into university and college. It was a total wash. We had one of the worst rain storms I can remember. So I came home early and disappointed and found my mom on the front porch. By that point, the rain had stopped and the sun was coming up. So I made the best of the situation and enjoyed one of my talks with my mother. Only this time, she listened and I talked about the start of my new chapter. I explained to her that I wanted to apply my gifts to helping people in need and proceeded to explain my four year plan. However, my mother did not share my enthusiasm. She was concerned that choosing this path would be too demanding and become a burden. After all, how rewarding could it be to listen to people's problems? Well, I was somewhat miffed that she did not give her blessing and I went in the house.

Mom continued to stay out on the porch and was joined by my dad. About an hour later, dad was calling me to come to the front door. He seemed in a panic and needed help getting my mother in the house. She was unable to walk, even with her cane and with his assistance. Dad and I carefully clutched each of her arms and practically carried her in. She was so frail. It was as if she had lost all motor control, so we gently placed her in the gold velour armchair with white trim, where she always sat. It was mom's favorite, French provincial style. It sounds tacky but in the 70's it was rather upscale. I hung on to the chair and the matching sofa for many years. I knew that if I reupholstered that chair, it would look fabulous, that shabby chic look. But it would always be the chair that my mother spent most of her dying days in and every time I looked at that chair, I saw her thin frail body.

One day I decided that it was time to let that memory go and so I made the call for the pick- up. But for now I see mom in her chair and by her expression, I could see that she was frightened too. She could barely speak and we thought that perhaps a good night sleep would do her good.

Mom had been sleeping on the main floor for some time. We had converted the dining room into the bedroom and dad stayed with mom downstairs. He slept most nights on the easy chair by mom's bed but there was nothing easy about his life at that time. I have to hand it to dad, he honored his vows and for better or worse, he was there for my mother. I remember on one occasion, dad had just reached his limit. To this day, I have no idea what the argument was about, but dad told mom that he couldn't do this anymore and that he was going to sleep upstairs and that she would have to fend for herself. My mother was crying and pleading with dad not to abandon her.

"I need your help" she cried. "I cannot do anything for myself anymore. This is what my life is now."

I heard my dad coming upstairs and I sat in my room not knowing what to do next. My brother John still lived at home but was working the night shift. Anyways he would not be able to do bathroom duty during the night or at any time. My mother had lost enough of her dignity. For the first time in my life, I was not angry with my father. He took care of her and did what he needed to do to give her comfort and support. But he needed some reprieve and a good night sleep. I didn't blame my mom either. She never asked for this. So I went downstairs and told mom that I would take over for dad and stay with her throughout the night. She seemed content with the new arrangement but did not want to be a burden on me either. I was in high school at the time and getting up early after a night of interrupted sleep was not easy. But that was nothing in comparison to what mom was going through. That one night lasted for about a week. Dad continued to take care of mom during the day while I was at school and my brother was at work and eventually dad went back to doing the night shift.

We had hoped that a good night sleep would have done mom some good, but she and dad were up most of the night. By Monday afternoon, mom was no longer verbal and we called the good doctor who quickly came to the home. He had given mom some meds for the pain, I think it was morphine and told us to keep her comfortable. Dr. R was a handsome dark haired man who I remember talking to often. He was so kind and gentle and I was trying to get an idea from him when mom might come out of her current state. Over the five years we had many setbacks and situations when we were sure this was the end. I remember coming home from school and not knowing if mom was going to still be alive. When I reflect back on that now, I think what a huge worry that was for a teenager. I guess when that is all you know, you just accept it for what it is. But after a few days mom would pull through. Perhaps this was one of those times? But this seemed different. Mom wasn't talking and she had this empty stare that I had never seen before. I knew what the answer would be, but I asked the doctor anyway, "Is this like one of the other times?" He took me aside and told me to prepare myself. He did not feel that mom was going to pull through this time. I thought that after five years of this living hell that I would have been prepared for those words, but I was not.

By this point we were still trying to accept the reality of this news and suddenly remembered that we were expecting my mother's relatives from Italy the following month. What were we going to do? I retreated to my room. I suppose that was another way of saying that I was trying to escape the reality that my mother's death was very near. I needed to find comfort within myself. We were a close family but we did not know how to talk to each other about what we were feeling. I remember my oldest brother Joe, coming up to my room and we talked about his relationship with mom in the early days. It was nice to hear stories of mom laughing and playing with her boy. He asked me to come downstairs and convince mom to eat so that she can build her strength. Apparently she had stopped eating. She was shutting down and her only way to communicate with us was to motion with her hand or moan. This was certainly a long way from the days when she would remind my sisters and me to speak the proper Italian. She did not like us to speak the dialect because it sounded rough and unsophisticated.

Mom insisted on being moved to every room in the house so my brothers and brother in laws did as she asked. They picked mom up in her golden velour chair and she toured the house. This was the home that my parents had built and mom had dreamed of her whole life. I had my own copy of Elizabeth Kubler -Ross that I had been reading in preparation for the end. I learned that this was a common request and that this would be mom's final tour of her home. I knew it was my role to advise my siblings of this part of the dying process. My knowledge and my insight was my gift.

Suddenly we heard an unexpected knock. I remember walking slowly down the hallway when I saw a woman's eyes peering through the small window of the door. She looked familiar but I knew that I had never met her before; neither had my sisters. We all approached the door to see who it was. Much to our disbelief, it was my mother's niece and her husband who had arrived one month earlier in hopes of surprising my mother. They were so excited but were not met with the same expression. We were in shock as mom was dying and we were in no condition to receive guests. Naturally we invited them in and explained the situation before we led them to see our ailing mother.

My mother's niece bore the same name as my mother but that was not all they had in common. I found myself staring at her often and could not believe her resemblance to mom. She had the same milky skin and dark brown eyes and I could see that she had the same zest for living that I am told mom had so long ago. She told us that she had noticed in the pictures that my mom had sent to her of the family that she was unwell, but had no idea that her condition was terminal. She was eager to see mom and reached out to embrace mom's tiny, fragile body. Unfortunately mom was unable to reciprocate or make eye contact with her, but she slowly raised her arm and pointed toward the table where she kept the picture of her niece. In a faint whisper mom said in Italian,

"I have been waiting for you".

We were all stunned and you could hear a pin drop. Mom had not spoken in nearly a week. Finally mom was reunited with her niece after all of these years. They sat there in silence as there were no words needed. Soon after, mom had motioned to her bed and there she remained. We had contacted our cousins and advised them of our unexpected guests. We also told them that mom was in her final stages of dying. They came to pay their respects to their much loved aunt and took the relatives with them. I remember that I found myself a quiet place to think and reflected upon the events of the afternoon. I thought about my mother's request the week before to clean out the dresser drawers. It was as if she knew she wouldn't have been able to ask this favor of me later. How did mom know that they would arrive earlier than expected and had she really been waiting for her loving niece to arrive?

Mom had been resting comfortably and her eyes were closed but her breathing was labored. My dad, sisters and I surrounded her bed. My brother John was tinkering in the basement. That was his way of keeping himself busy and my other brothers had gone home for a while to be with their wives and children. I remember lying on the bed beside mom and we were all quiet listening for her breath as we knew what it meant when we would no longer hear it. We had a few moments of panic but they were false alarms. I remember whispering in mom's ear knowing full well that she likely couldn't hear me, but I told her that it was okay for her to go. Dad and Josie sat right in front of mom and caught a bit of saliva that came up when she took her last breath. Tina was at mom's feet and I was still lying beside her. I heard dad gasp and call out her name while Josie and Tina cried. I knew that God had taken her in his arms. The rest is still a blur but I remember going to find my brother John in the basement and the two of us ended up crying in the cold cellar. We had lived with mom's cancer for five years and had many close calls, yet when she died, we were unprepared and went into shock. I had never known anyone who had died before my mother.

My mom's funeral was the very first funeral that I had ever been to. The whole experience felt very unreal. We had the funeral on the Tuesday because of the long weekend and then the following week, I began my first year at university. It was definitely a new chapter only not the one I had anticipated. My mother's death had a huge impact on my life. Most of the time especially within that first year, I felt numb. People would often ask me what I was feeling and would look at me strangely when I would answer, nothing. I actually felt nothing. People stopped asking after a while.

Chapter 29

A Motherless Daughter

MY LIFE as a motherless daughter had begun. I was nineteen years old. I felt sad and alone on that big campus and really felt that I belonged to no one. I remember coming home after a long day at school, calling out, "mom I'm home" as I had done so many times before. I was strangely expecting her to call back, "I 'm in here". Yet I knew that she wouldn't. I remember running from room to room looking for her like I was some crazy person, totally out of touch with reality. But when that reality finally sunk in, I cried and cried for hours and hours. Mom did not live here anymore. Mom was gone. So much had changed in my life and I didn't feel like myself anymore. I felt like a different person. I didn't even know who that person was, but I knew that something inside of me had died too.

Caring for a loved one with cancer for five years took a huge toll on the whole family. Every ones lives were focused on the dying member. My two oldest brothers had lived away from the family home with their families for a long time, and my sisters were both newly married. My brother John and I remained at home with my parents. At the age of fifteen, I was adjusting to living at home without my sisters and literally over the period of a few short months, I was cleaning a large two- story, four bedroom house doing laundry and anything else that was asked of me. Then a year later at sixteen, I started to drive because someone had to take dad for groceries and other errands. It was a full schedule and there were not a lot of other kids my age doing what I was doing. It was a struggle and there were times when I resented all of these responsibilities. But I knew that my mom was appreciative. She would always give me praise and encouragement and then cry and tell me how sorry she was that she couldn't do any of the chores that she felt a mother should do. I suppose she felt haunted by her own past, thinking how she felt having to quit school and take on the chores for her mother. Only I continued to attend school and rarely resented my mother for being in this situation. How could I fault her? She was living in her own hell. My dad on the other hand was not sympathetic of my situation and frankly I was not always of his either. He was often so angry and needed to control everyone and everything. I knew that he was angry that his wife had this horrible disease called cancer and his retirement years had been spent caring for her. He knew that someday, she would die and leave him all alone. After all, who knows more about abandonment than dad? I did not know it then, but I understand now that dad's anger was really about his fear. My mother's illness took such a toll on us all. Dad was often agitated and I found myself involved in arguments with him daily with mom as our buffer. I felt criticized and controlled by him. I needed to answer to him for everything. If I was heading into the garage, he needed to know what I needed from there. If I was going downstairs to do the laundry and he felt it was too late in the evening to do it, he showed his disapproval. In dad's eyes, I couldn't do anything right.

My duties continued long after my mother died and this created even more resentment and tension in my relationship with my father. As I grew older and into my twenties, I felt that I had earned the right to have my own independence. But that was a constant struggle with my father. He had a difficult time of letting go and giving me my freedom. The more he yelled, the more I felt I had to stand up for myself. All I wanted was to feel happiness again and find the person in me that I felt I had lost. I was searching for myself. I felt I had lost so much that I wanted to feel alive and energetic. But my father misinterpreted this energy. I never felt validated by him. I allowed him to make me feel like I was a bad person doing bad things, even though I knew I was doing nothing wrong. Once mom had died, I felt like I was living in a prison and I knew that I could not continue to live my life under those conditions. Dad's temper was becoming more explosive and it was difficult to figure out what would trigger him. He had become so unpredictable and I was frightened to be at home with him. I had made a decision to move away from my father's house. I knew that this was not going to be easy for my father to accept. In the Italian culture, moving out of the family home before marriage is considered a slap in the face. Dad had been a good provider all of his life and would not understand my desire to leave in search of personal fulfillment. He had provided a roof over my head, food to eat and a warm bed to sleep. At twenty-four years old, I had finished university and was working in my field. I felt that if I tried to explain to him my feelings, the impact that mom's death had on me and the reasons why I needed to go, then perhaps he would understand and give me his blessing. Unfortunately, my father became outraged and advised me that if I left his house, that I could never come back. Despite feeling devastated and more alone than I had ever felt in my life, I had to go. I know now that my father felt that I was abandoning him and the family. He had lost my mother five years before and now he felt that he was losing me too. Yet I too was feeling abandoned by the only parent that I had left. My brother John understood what I was feeling and did his best to support me. But I knew that he also felt a loyalty to dad. Other family members felt an even greater loyalty to my father and I knew that we were no longer working together as a family. We were divided. Up until the day that I left, the arguments continued between us and mom was no longer there to comfort me. In fact no one was except for Josie. I remember when I went to see Josie to tell her that I told dad I was moving out. She was folding laundry and said

"I don't necessarily agree with everything that you are doing, but I will stand by you". She made her position known to the family as well and I will be forever grateful to her for taking that stand and defending my honor.

Chapter 30

April Showers Bring May Flowers

SPRINGTIME WAS always such a pleasant time growing up. It seemed that in those days, spring weather actually occurred in the spring. I don't ever remember it being cold or rainy on Easter when I was a young girl. It was always perfect weather for wearing our new floral dresses, sun hats and white gloves. My sisters and I would walk to church with our parents, dad in his suit and mom with one of her dresses that was made especially for her. Although mom made us wear hats, she was really the only one of us who looked good in them. My mother had a love of hats and wore them well. It was a time when chocolate actually smelled and tasted like real chocolate and the lamb my parents served for Easter dinner was fresh. I mean really fresh. Our houses were small but somehow there was a place for everyone at the table. I hold a lot of these memories close to my heart and at times long for those days when we were all together. Thank goodness for home movies when we need to be reminded that there were actually happier times than what we were going through in the spring of 1995. This would be a springtime that we would never forget for the rest of all our lives. Everything was changing and there was nothing that we could do about it.

On April 11 1995 I wrote:

I cannot believe that I have not written in so long. I am shocked at how quickly the time has gone by. So much has happened and I have so much to tell. I have not been working since March. It is a long unimportant story but basically, we all got laid off and I received a severance package. So I have been home and it has been great because Josie and I have had a new adventure every day. I thought I would be able to sleep during these last few months of my pregnancy before experiencing the sleepless nights with a newborn. No way. Josie phones me every morning at nine am and asks, "So what do you want to do today?" Every day is an adventure with Josie and she is always so much fun. I can never say no to Josie and I haul my pregnant ass up the mountain to her place. A quick cup of tea and some baked goods of course and off we go. Josie and I have gone shopping and out for lunch. We've done some crazy things like try on hats, all kinds of hats which we both look hilarious in. Even as adults, we still don't wear hats well. We laugh at ourselves until we pee a little in our pants. I love being with her. We also bought some things for the baby. Josie bought this lovely white knit outfit. It will be perfect for the baptism when we take off the baby's gown. Josie came down with the kids and helped paint the baby's room. It looks so beautiful. She is a great painter especially with that trim work. It's that attention to detail. But in these past few weeks, Josie seems to have taken a turn. She has had some difficulty passing stool. She has had a cat scan which shows a thickening of the lining of the rectum. She needs to go for a barium test. I am frightened for her. How much more does she have to go through? We are all scared. Josie is looking weaker and even more frail. She hasn't been able to eat much because she can't have a bowel movement. She doesn't want anyone to know. I have so many feelings inside me that I cannot articulate. I just keep remembering that it was only a month ago that we were out together having a great time. Is it all coming to an end? Oh my dear god what is to happen to my beautiful Josie?

On April 13/95 Josie wrote:

Even though all my tests came back clean at the end of January, here I am writing again. My worst fear is back. Cat scan confirmed cancer has returned to my rectum and pelvic area. Dr. C called tonight and wants me in hospital Tuesday 18th 8:00am. He's not sure if I'll make it till then w/o having a bowel movement. Should severe cramping occur call him ASAP at home. Otherwise he will operate Tues. He plans to perform a complete hysterectomy and colostomy. God please help me fight this disease and win.

Sunday April 23 1995 I wrote:

Josie had surgery at 10:00am today and at 10:35 am Dr. C came in to the waiting area and told us that-it wasn't good. They couldn't even do what they had intended whatever that was. There was too much in the pelvic area. This linitus plastica has spread everywhere; the abdominal wall, the liver everywhere, the colon and the bowel. Oh my dear God. He suggested that chemotherapy would not help at this point. Josie has an untreatable cancer and he said that she will go downhill from here. What does this mean for Josie? Is she going to die? I can't bear this, it is too painful. I feel like I want to die too, but I have this beautiful new life growing inside of me. Josie has something horrible growing inside of her that is killing her. I remember Josie saying to me that our situation was so ironic. I understand now what she was meaning. In three weeks I will give birth to my first child. What will happen to Josie?

Recently, I was talking to my sister Tina about this very point in time following Josie's surgery. She reminded me of my phone call to her from the hospital. She stated that I was totally hysterical when I called her to tell her of Dr. C's latest prognosis. Tina remembers that I was completely out of control and out of my mind like she had never seen or heard me before. I was initially shocked to hear this because I had not remembered this at all. I know that when I read that journal entry from that day, there is an ache in my stomach even now, that I can't put words to. Those raw emotions are familiar to me but I realize how much of that deep pain has been blocked to the point that I forgot this moment of temporary insanity. I am sure that I am not alone. It does pose a very important question and that is, where does all that forgotten raw emotion go? I need to really think about that one.

Chapter 31

Saying Our Final Goodbyes

May 10, 1995 at 8:43 am I wrote:

I am lying in bed thinking about Josie. Things are unbelievable and unbearable. Since she came home on April 28 1995 from the hospital, my wedding anniversary, she seems to have not improved. Josie has lost more weight. We have tried many alternatives and homeopathic remedies but Josie had some complications and has little appetite. I feel like she is slipping away but then she appears hopeful. I was there yesterday on Tuesday and I had not seen her since Saturday. Andrea had a dance recital and Josie went too. I've been told by Dr. R that I can't go there every day anymore because it is too much for me and he says that he is worried about my energy level and how prepared I will be for the delivery. Josie understands. I explained it to her but I was there yesterday and it was just the two of us. It was so nice because we talked. That is what we do best. She told me that everyone is hyper and forcing her to eat; even people's voices are bothering her. She said that the only person not getting on her nerves was me because my voice is so soothing. I felt special when she said that but did come to the defense of others. I tried to explain that everyone loves and cares for her so much that they want her to eat and gain strength. Josie told me that it is easy for her to slip away right now especially when she is in pain. She went to a Native Indian naturalist with John this morning. She said that she was disappointed because she gave her essiac which she has already been taking. But she said that it tastes different and should not be diluted. Has she been taking it wrong all this time?

She asked me how the children are doing so I told her the truth. Josie appreciates that. I told her that Anthony seems frightened and afraid that she will die. Paul hasn't said too much but I feel he is confused and Andrea is withdrawing too and told me that she feels sad. It is such a sad situation because Josie has always been such an attentive mother, an excellent mother.

Later on in the day as I was getting ready to leave, Josie asked me to never abandon the kids. She wants me to be there for her children especially Andrea because I understand her. I promised her that I would never abandon them and that she has been a wonderful mother. I will always try to do for them what she would have done.

Josie told me that she is very sorry that she cannot be here for me and the baby. She stated that she has tried but cannot do it. I told her that it wasn't her fault. She has always been there for me. She asked that although Tina and I are named for the children, she wants Chiara involved and Franca to take Andrea from time to time to be with the girls. I told her that I would tell them that. She asked that Chris be there for John and the boys. She told me to have dad change the will so that her share goes to John and the kids. She wants me to make sure that John pays off credit cards and mortgage.

"There is the life insurance too". I felt like we were saying goodbye. I gave her a kiss on the cheek and told her I loved her. It was late and I had to go home but I didn't want to leave her. As I got to the step on the front porch, she asked John to call me back in. She said to me,

"Sal if there is a way I can come back to you, I will."

She smiled and I smiled back and told her that I would like that. I kissed her again and I left, only to feel like I would never see my sister again. I cried my heart out the whole way home and pleaded with God not to take her away from us. Could this really be happening? What kind of a God would allow our family to be destroyed? Who in God's name is going to love and care for her children as much as she does? I felt such anguish and pain pouring out of my heart. I have tried to be so strong for Josie, the kids, the family and my unborn baby. I feel so torn with my feelings. I am on the brink of losing the one person that means so much to me and at the same time, ready to give life to my first born child. This is absolutely crazy. I feel crazy. My whole life these past months feels insane. I feel guilty too; guilty for not feeling the joy that a first time pregnancy brings and guilty that I have moments of happiness when I think of being a new mom. Then I ask myself," How can I feel such happiness when my sister is in so much pain and ready to die? My heart was pounding and my screams were getting louder and louder. Tears were gushing out of my eyes that I couldn't see out my windshield. I was angry and I let *him* know that there was not one damn good reason for all of this to be happening. No good would ever come out of this. NEVER My heart was breaking and all I could think of was her three babies and how they were going to live their lives without their mother in it. I know what is ahead for them as I have lived it. The little girl in me still misses my mother and now I will have to live without Josie too. I feel so alone already.

I knew that I should probably pull over but I didn't. I felt so out of control behind this wheel and in my life. Everything was changing and there wasn't a thing I could do about it. I was getting closer to my home when all of a sudden I felt a sense of calm and my hysterics suddenly came to an end. It was the most exhausting drive I have ever had but I was home. I came home to Chris' open arms and we talked. I told him that my sister and I had said our goodbyes. I had never seen that look on his face before. He was so sad. Chris loved Josie too.

I had Dad, Tina and John's phone calls to return so I did that. I told Tina about my talk with Josie and suggested to her that she have some quiet time with Josie tomorrow. In my mind I was thinking oh my God is there going to be a tomorrow? At about 10:30 pm the phone rang and my heart stopped. It was John. Josie asked him to call me to tell me that she vomited. Josie is incapable of vomiting but somehow she did after she had her essiac. I was happy and I thought once again that there was hope and she was going to beat this disease. The vomit was mucus; stringy and brown. I was convinced that this vomit was the ugly cancer that was filling up my beautiful sister's body.

I slept through the night. I think I was just so exhausted. I had hoped that when I woke up, the nightmare would be over. But the next morning, little had changed. In fact, John phoned me to say that he was taking Josie to the hospital to receive intravenous. Josie is weaker than yesterday. She can't drink now so the fear of dehydration is near. I think her death is near too. I spoke with all three of my brothers this morning. Joe and I had a really important conversation and we talked about his son's upcoming wedding. John and I spoke the way we always do and Sammy was brief. He seemed to try to hide his feelings. Dad, well he just cries all the time now. He is on his way out too and I know that at eighty two years old, he wishes that he could trade places with his young beautiful daughter. I am not sure where life is going. Everything we have known has changed and will never be the same. I hope that I can have the strength to take care of my baby and give Josie's kids all the love they need. I have made that promise and I intend to keep it. There is so much I want to say, maybe on another day. Josie and John should be at the hospital by now receiving the intravenous. I hope she will come home tomorrow. I hope Tina has a chance to talk with Josie too.

The family has been very supportive of me regarding the baby. I have really tried to hold it together because I don't want my baby to suffer any defects, but it's getting harder and harder. Dr. R said the heartbeat is strong and regular. I hope the baby is not distressed or colic as a result of all the stress that I have been experiencing throughout my whole pregnancy. I had asked Josie to baptize the baby. She is convinced that the baby is a Nicole but I am not sure. I hope Josie gets to see Nicole or Mitchell. I had a dream last night of a baby boy who was happy and he had the biggest blue eyes I've ever seen. So I am thinking it's a boy.

What a month. We have a birth, a wedding and pending death. I just don't know in what order. Everything is changing, but my love for Josie will always stay the same. My sister has

become the mother I lost and the friend that I
trust the most.

Chapter 32

Room # 608

On May 10, 1995 at 10:12pm I wrote:

Josie was admitted to hospital today. She has been hooked up to the IV and is receiving some nourishment now. So much has happened today. So much has been said amongst all of us. I arrived at the hospital this afternoon and everyone else arrived into the late afternoon and evening. Our brothers and sister in laws were all there too. I have had a lot of opportunity to talk with Josie further about what she said and what she wants. She doesn't feel that she will make it for the baby's delivery but she will try to hang on. She says she would like to be the baby's spirit. Neither of us really knows what that means. Josie always said the baby was a girl but now she is rethinking her prediction given my dream of little blue eyes. She suggested that Tina take her place and baptize the baby. She wants us all to be there for Al's wedding and be there in support of our brother. She also gave us a list of her wants. She wants to wear her red suit with the lace and long sleeves. She doesn't want us to wait too long to be rid of her clothes. She'd like us to give them away and wants some of her fancy things to be put away in a trunk so that Andrea can play dress up. Her costume jewelry is for dress up but she wants the real jewelry to be put away for the children. She was also very clear that she wants any monetary donations to go to homeless children. Nancy is to finish the baby blanket that she crocheted. I was willing to bring my baby home in it with one row missing, but Josie wouldn't have it. She has spoken with Nancy about finishing it. Josie expressed her concern about her children coming home to an empty house after school until John gets home from work. We can manage as a lot of us will help. It was a very emotional time for us all. Josie seemed so calm as she delegated. Dad was tearful and almost pleading with Josie. He asked her who would now take him to do groceries and his banking, as they have done together for several years. Josie suggested that I would take over this responsibility as I will now be at home during the day with the new baby. I can't remember any of her other requests. I think this was it. In terms of my feelings, I don't have any right now.

On May 13th 1995 Tina wrote:

Today is Saturday and I am here at St. Joseph hospital. Sam was here a bit to keep me company while I am taking care of Josie. I sent

John home for a shower and change. I have been here every day (all day) since Thursday May 11th. I cannot leave her. I have to be with her. I just washed her with Nurse Kathleen and used Lauren powder. She has been wonderful with Josie.

Josie is getting weaker; so much worse than last night. I am afraid that her time is coming near. She is comfortable with the new pain medication that Dr. M prescribed on Friday. The nausea has stopped at least. Dr. C came in this a.m. He kissed Josie on her forehead. He turned all red and was almost in tears. He left quickly. I am sure it was very difficult for him to see her like this too. As rough as he is and lacking in bedside manner with the families of the patients, Josie liked him and would often say that they had an understanding. I still cannot give up on Jos. I love her so much. My twin soul mate. I still pray the rosary each day and hope for that "thimble of help from God" that Fr. Peter spoke with us about at school. I am being realistic but yet I still have hope. I can't let go. This is a nightmare. I go to sleep at night to get away from it and I hope that when I awake that the nightmare would be over, but it is still there. Dad and my brothers are here every day and so is John and his sister, Chiara. All five children were at Sal's Friday night for a sleep over. She is planting flowers with them on Saturday morning. John's brother Midge and Nancy will pick up Josie's kids on Saturday night and keep them for the rest of the weekend. Tomorrow is Mother's Day.

I hope that Josie will make it until then for the kids, especially Paul. He made her something special at school. Sal and Chris' baby is due on May 18th and Al and Rosie's wedding is on the 20th. I don't know what will happen this week where Josie is concerned.

I can't believe it!!!! Josie told me to put her housecoat on and she took a walk to the elevators and back to her room at 608. She got back into bed and said "I am exhausted. I want to sleep". John is so wonderful; he won't leave Josie's side for a second.

At 4:20pm Josie makes me change her pjs. The new set we put on this am were, " too bulky" she said. So we changed them. She is happy now.

I am sitting here quietly watching Josie sleep. I know that she is frail now, pale too but I still see the same beautiful precious and wonderful girl that I grew up with. The sweetheart that I have shared so many private thoughts with for such precious and few years. It's so hard to believe and accept that I'm going to lose her now so very young. She will be 40 this July 1995. Oh Lord why my soul mate?

Pm. Saturday May 13th 1995 Tina wrote:

Josie is having a rough night. The end is near. I take daddy home at 8:00pm. My brothers go home too. Sal and Chris remain at the hospital with John and Chiara. Joey was there too. I get home and I can't rest. In my stomach I feel such pain. I go back to the hospital with Rocky and take the kids to Clare's for the night. The time is drawing closer. We all spend the night with John and Josie and we all have the same feeling. The time is here. We took turns with John in room 608. She kept sitting up in bed to hug John. At one point, he got into bed with her to comfort her. Chiara was with them but then she ran into the lounge to get us. Sal and I rushed into the room and saw Josie staring up at John and up at the wall. She took a last breath and at 4:55 am and then she was gone. The angels came for her and her spirit went to heaven.

May 14, 1995 I wrote:

It's 6:20am and it is Mother's Day and Josie just died at five minutes to five am today. I am sitting in her room #608 and she is lying there. I need some time to myself, some time to reflect on what has just happened. I feel numb. It was a terrible night of unrest for Josie. She was so restless up and down, moving around, struggling with death not wanting to go but yet knowing she had to. John has been remarkable and has stayed by her side all night long. She died in his arms. Tina, Chiara and I were with him when Josie opened her eyes wide, looked up and took her last breath. What a tragic day it is. One, we cannot ever forget and a Mother's Day that cannot be celebrated for many years to come. Josie died on Mother's Day and she was one of the greatest mothers I've ever known. How could I ever thank her for all her kindness and generosity, guidance and support? I can be there for her three beautiful children. They are now motherless but they have a wonderful father, many loving aunts and uncles from both sides of the family, and the privilege of having one of the world's greatest mother. I miss her already and I will remember her and keep her memory alive. God Bless you Josie. I am waiting for you!

On Sunday May 14th Tina wrote:

It's Mother's Day and Josie has joined mom in heaven after thirteen and a half years since her death. She looked the most like mom too. We went to the funeral home to make the arrangements and by 9:30 am, John, Sal and I and our mates went to John's brother's house to tell the children. They cried and we all cried. It was so difficult. Sal and Chris took the kids home with them until Monday night when Josie is laid out.

Chapter 33

The Funeral

On May 18th 1995 I wrote:

Today is my due date. I have had a lot of physical pain for most of the night and morning. I hope the baby gives me a break because I need a few days to relax before the big delivery. I am sure that Josie will orchestrate something that will work in my favor. Her funeral was yesterday and visitation and last respects started on Monday evening. What a tribute. There were so many people and so much support for our family. People were sharing their sorrow and comforting one another, I have never seen so many grown men cry. I think Josie herself was surprised that she had such an impact on so many people. Death is always a sad occasion but this death was truly tragic. When someone as young and loving and as beautiful as Josie, dies, it is a tragedy. It is like a devastation that hit all who have ever known and loved her and they were there to pay their last respects to her. The line ups were long and as crazy as this sounds, I felt that I too was consoling the people who were coming through the reception line just as much as they were comforting me. Everyone was truly touched by Josie and many will feel her loss.

There were times when I felt that we were just going through the motions. I remember my sister, Tina who rarely takes anything, had a little help to get her through this emotional ordeal. I being nine months pregnant and ready to deliver, literally any day now, couldn't take a thing. I remember so many people looking at me and I knew what they were thinking, "My god she is so pregnant," but mostly they were sad for me. Many of Josie's dearest friends knew how much she meant to me and how much I meant to her. Many of them came up to me and told me things that I didn't even know that they knew about me. They told me that Josie talked about me all the time. Wow, imagine how special that made me feel? I was thinking, who would be proud of me now? Josie died and all my secrets have gone with her. How can she ever be replaced? I was already feeling alone and abandoned, but I couldn't think of all that now. There were people still coming in droves and we were all there to receive them.

Dad, what is there to say about dad? He was an eighty two year old man who had been abandoned by his parents through death at a very young age. He worked the farms and fell in love with my mother who in her own strange way, loved him for over forty years. He moved what family they had at that time to Canada, had more kids, worked some more and made a lot of sacrifices as he used to tell us for the family. All to one day lose his wife, whom he adored and now he loses his beloved daughter who is only thirty nine years old.

Where the hell is the justice in that? I remember dad often willing himself to die so that he could take Josie's place. As a parent now, I get that. I remember him telling me that he was Paul's age when his own mother died. I am sure that the child within him was grieving his mother loss all over again. But there he sat in the reception line right next to his daughter receiving everyone's condolences. Dad maintained his honor and pride and showed strength for the family. We were all looking out for dad. After all suffering this kind of trauma at his age, we were worried about him. We were all looking after each other and we all took turns at being strong. We are a family who has had our fair share of tragedy, and in the end, there is a lot of love among us. John's family was a huge help. They loved Josie like she was their own sister and got the children ready for the visitation. I still picture all three of them going up to the casket with their Mother's Day gifts in hand; their mother laying there in her bright red suit with the lace on the sleeves just as she had requested four days earlier. What they must have been feeling? I remember standing with them admiring their mother's beauty. I don't think they knew what to think. They didn't know what was ahead of them. They didn't know that they would feel a longing for their mother for the rest of their lives. They didn't know that her death was the beginning of a void that can never be filled by anyone else.

We found an envelope tucked inside Josie's journal on her bedside. Among other things she had left instructions that she did not want an open casket. She was concerned and did not want people to "gawk" at her. Those were her precise words. There is something that I have not really mentioned about Josie and that is that she was incredibly vain. Although she was a natural beauty, she was very conscientious about her appearance. She loved clothes and shoes and jewelry and nice smelly perfumes. In a nut shell she was a real girly girl.

But over the last months she had become ashamed of her appearance. She knew how much she had deteriorated and how much this cancer had taken from her. So I understood her reluctance to be displayed amongst all of us to "gawk" as she would say. John did too, but he didn't agree with her decision. He knew how Josie had deteriorated too. It was obvious to all of us, but to him, she was a beauty to the end. And so he insisted on the open casket and I am glad that he did. It was actually quite comforting to know that each morning we would wake and go down to the funeral home to see Josie. The funeral guys did a great job on her prep and she looked exactly like the Josie we all knew and loved ten months ago before this whole nightmare began. In a weird kind of way, I looked forward to looking at her in the casket and carrying on our little conversations. At least I could see her and touch her.

Unfortunately all great things come to an end, and of course I mean that sarcastically. We were faced with the final day which meant the closing of the casket and the actual funeral, ceremony, mass etc. I remember looking and touching our red laced beauty and saying my last good- byes. It felt surreal. Was this really the end? How can you say good bye to someone who has been so much a part of your life. My pain was so deep. I remember trying to be strong but I couldn't hold back my tears. In fact, I couldn't even breathe. It all seemed too final and I just couldn't leave her there. But I knew that we had to. I knew what was happening but I still didn't believe that it was happening to us. Tina felt the same way. Several years later, Tina told me that after the wake when everyone left, she was thinking of calling Josie to discuss the day's events. We both smiled and admitted that even now after all of these years, we still catch ourselves feeling that way.

The rest of the day was a complete blur with only bits and pieces of our memories. We all went back to Tina's house where her close friends had prepared a lovely reception. It was very kind of them. I know that they did it for Tina but they loved Josie too. Everybody did. The house was full of family and friends whose hearts were bleeding for us all. We were all thinking of Josie's three gentle angels and why they have to live the rest of their lives without their mother; especially when they had the best. I tried to be social but I did not have much left in me. I think I was topped up. We had just buried Josie and now we had a family wedding in a few days. Somewhere in all of this, Chris and I were having our first child and I knew that childbirth was not going to be easy. There was so much to think about but I couldn't think and I couldn't feel. I needed to rest and that is what I did.

Chapter 34

Let My Babies Cry

IT IS unimaginable that such a young beautiful woman in her prime could have her life threatened by such a deadly disease. It is unbelievable that after giving your heart and your soul to your children, that you are ripped right out of their lives. It is unjust that innocent children who have been brought into this world and loved by a mother may never remember what it's like to feel her touch. Anthony, Paul and Andrea were three little angels picked by God to endure the pain of mother loss. Only they did not know it until their mother was gone. How can we explain to children that the mother that waited for them to come home every day after school was no longer going to be waiting there for them? Or how do you explain to them that the sad feeling they feel inside will take a long time to go away? Or how do you even explain why mommy had to die? Dealing with the answers to all these questions when you are an adult is hard enough because we don't understand it ourselves. But helping a child make sense of it all, sounds nearly impossible. Do we sign them up for therapy and hope that they can pour their hearts out to a stranger, or do we keep it within the family. After all, who wants the best for them more than family? Maybe the solution is to find them a new mommy and hope for the best. Or maybe we can just let them cry. That is what Josie wanted for her children.

In that note we found on Josie's night table just after she died read:

My wishes for Tina and Sal.

Never forget my babies. They are so sensitive and gentle. Always talk about me to them. Don't let them repress their tears. They must cry.

And with these three simple words, Josie gave her children permission to let out their pain and release their tears. But what happens when you cannot cry or when the pain is so overwhelming? Many lash out and express anger because that is the only emotion that they can understand. What happens to all the fear, the unanswered questions and the loss of your voice when you feel that no one is listening? What do you do when everything you know about your life has now changed and you don't know how to get it back? What happens to all these raw emotions? Where do they all go? Is Josie right? Will crying help them to heal their broken hearts? I think it is a start. Josie always knew what her babies needed. I know that she thought of them and how they would cope with this terrible tragedy. Imagine her fear and anguish knowing that she had to leave them. We learned from Josie's journal entries that she was a strong woman who showed a lot of courage by carrying on and doing what she did best for her children and her family during those last ten months of her life. Of course she was fearful who wouldn't be, and I am sure that when she was alone in her home, she cried too.

Chapter 35

The Wedding

DING DONG Wedding bells are ringing. Can you believe we have gone from the most horrific thing that can happen to a family to my brother Joe's oldest son's marriage? All of this within the week. Thank God for my sister Tina. She made sure that not only her children, but Josie's children were all set and dressed for the wedding. It was enough that I had to roll my pregnant ass out of bed. It was May 20th. Josie's funeral was three days ago and I was due to delivery this baby two days ago. Chris was so worried for me and the baby. He knew I wanted to keep my promise to Josie and support our brother in his son's wedding, but he was convinced that it was too risky. I insisted and anyways a promise is a promise. So we put the all ready hospital suit case in the trunk of the car and drove off to the big city.

The wedding was beautiful. It was a fabulous hall with gorgeous crystal chandeliers. It was very glamorous and upscale and I remember thinking that this was the first wedding without Josie. I knew that it was the beginning of a lot of first without Josie. I remember Tina and I couldn't even look at each other. We were just doing what we had to do to get through it. All the children were excited to be together at a family wedding. I remember I was wearing a black skirt and a beautiful mauve top with white magnolias that a friend had lent me. It was beautiful but I would only wear these big flowers as a maternity top. It looked great with my dark hair and it was the dressiest thing I had that fit. Let's just say I wasn't looking as glamorous as the venue and I certainly wasn't feeling as sparkly as the chandeliers. There was no sense in getting something new at this point in the pregnancy and anyways, not much time and energy to be shopping around in the malls. So there we are at the wedding in my outfit and of course my signature white sandals. My feet and ankles were so swollen; it was the only shoe that would fit me. Chris looked very handsome in his suit despite the look on his face and the keys in his hand. He was ready to get back into the car and straight to the delivery room. We all tried to make the best of the situation. As hard as this day was for all of us, I can't imagine what it must have been like for my brother, Joe and his wife, Doris. I know that they were touched by all of the family's support and they knew that Josie had not only given her blessing but her orders for all of us to be there. The joy of celebrating their son's wedding will be marked by such a sad event. My oldest brother Joe is perhaps the most sensitive of all three brothers. It is actually sweet to see. But that day, Joe needed to be strong and although he had a few moments where he had trouble holding it together, he stayed strong, for his son, for all of us and for Josie.

Chapter 36

The Delivery

WE HAD survived another one of the life changing events in the family. We made the trek along the highway back to our home safe and sound. I know Chris was relieved. By 2:00 am we were tucked in bed totally exhausted. Naturally it didn't take Chris long to fall asleep. For someone who was worried that we were going to deliver the baby at the reception hall, he certainly wasted no time falling into a deep sleep. Me on the other hand, I was wide awake. I didn't feel right and I didn't know why. I tried to convince myself that my fatigue, not to mention everything else that had happened this week, was the reason for this uneasiness. Maybe tonight was the night that I would have this baby. Is this why I am feeling so different? Josie would know. I should call her I thought to myself. She would know for sure. She has had three kids, she knows but it is so late. I can't phone her now. I will wake up the whole household. I really tried to force myself to sleep and tossed and turned for a while. And then it hit me. I can't pick up the phone anymore. She cannot answer me. She is gone and I must figure this out on my own. I think that this was the first realization that she was not there for me. I felt very sad and alone. After a really good cry I pleaded with whoever

153

would listen and asked for a few hours of sleep at least. It was 4:30 am and I knew that the next big event in this family was having the baby and I needed to be as ready as possible. By the grace of God, someone heard me and the next time I looked at the clock, it was 6:30 am. I woke up to feeling pain down below and felt the urge to pee only to discover a show of blood. I think that this is the mucus plug that they talk about in all the books. I wish I knew what to do. I wish I could call my sister Tina but she wouldn't appreciate a call this early in the morning after a long day and evening at the wedding. And anyways, we just didn't have that kind of relationship at that time. I thought to myself I must rely on my husband, after all we are in this together. Trying to wake Chris up from a deep sleep is like ... I don't know what, it's just not easy. So I nudged and pushed and got louder and then pop, he was up asking if everything was okay. We lay there together and I told him about my night and the two hours of sleep that I got. I told Chris that I thought I was going into labor. So we started to time the contractions and pulled out the baby books that we had been reading all along. Finally the contractions were at five minute intervals. So we called Dr. M at about 10:00 am. It is now Sunday the 21st and he suggested we go down to the hospital and he would meet us there. What a guy! Since our bags were already in the car, we were all ready to go. So we get there and sure enough the doctor is there and he examines me. I tell him about the plug and the show and he asks me if my water broke. I told him that I didn't know but that I have been peeing a lot. So much for all those baby books I had been reading! The nurses attached me to a fetal monitor and said that the baby was fine. I was very relieved to hear that after such a stressful pregnancy. I was continuing to have contraction and was rather proud of the fact that I was handling it all. I thought to myself that these contractions are not as bad as everyone has made them out to be. I must have a very high pain tolerance. After all, everything I have been through in a week, I was numb. The nursing staff was wonderful and they confirmed that I was in the early stages of labor. They decided that it would be best if I went home and rested more comfortably there. So reluctantly, I bent over to pull on my elastic waist maternity stretch pants and then it happened. My water broke and all this water came gushing down my legs and everywhere. It just kept coming out so I tried to sit on the bed to stop it. Chris and I were amazed. The nurses came running in and changed the bed and Dr. M came running in too. Everyone was there and little did I know at that time that this event marked the beginning of my loss of dignity forever. My water had broken and I was in true labor. The contractions were unbearable. This is what everyone has been talking about.

They moved us into a birthing room at 11:00 am and the contractions kept coming. Chris was a fabulous coach. We had a room with a Jacuzzi tub and I went in it as it is supposed to be comforting. But by 3:00pm, nothing was quite that comforting and so I had asked for the epidural. The anesthesiologist arrived and the epidural was in. It was very difficult to hold still while I was having contractions but I hung on to Chris and we got through it. Immediately after the epidural I felt relief and then really itchy. What the hell was this itch? I just needed to relax. I was told that some people have a reaction so they gave me something for the itch. I don't know what but whatever it was, it put me right to sleep and I slept for a long time after.

According to Chris I was sleeping right through some really intense contractions and apparently I did not even flinch. Chris was getting worried but I was getting the best sleep that I had ever had in months. They kept topping me up and I kept sleeping. The doctor and the nurses would be checking me periodically to see how many centimeters I had dilated. I would just fall right back to sleep but at 11:15pm on Sunday night, Dr. M announced that I was now 10cm and that it was time to push. Push. I didn't even want to wake up. I was in such a deep comfortable sleep. But they propped me up and told me to bear down and feel it in my crotch. Well we had a problem already. I was not even feeling my crotch and so we had to wait for the epidural to wear off. It was now midnight and I was propped up again and I had to push. What a challenge this was. I felt so conflicted as I knew it would not be long before I became a new mother. But all I wanted at that time was to have the comfort of my own. But it wasn't just mom that I was longing for. It had been so long since she was in my life. I wanted Josie to be there too holding my other hand. I prayed that she would help me and give me the strength to see this through. I did not realize that this process of pushing was going to take another hour and a half. But it did. Surprisingly, I stayed very calm and that meant that I did not yell, or scream obscenities at my husband. He thought for sure I would be that type. All of that would have been difficult especially since I was vomiting the whole time that I was pushing. Basically I felt like I was going on both ends if you know what I mean. Most women unfortunately do. I was however becoming somewhat frustrated as I felt that whenever I was making gains and pushing baby out , it would slide back in. This happened quite a few times and I was getting more and more exhausted. As a result, I ended up tearing to the left and was also cut so that the baby's head could come through. I did not have the strength to push this baby out so they had to get the vacuum to suction it out. I thought great, let the vacuum do this but no I still had to push. I tried to negotiate with the hospital staff and told them in the nicest way that I could no longer push this baby out and that they had to find another way. Chris had been so supportive all along. He knew what I had been through, but out of nowhere he grabs my arm and says,

"Listen it's time to push this baby out. Now push".

I had been with Chris for nine years and never had he taken this tone with me. I could have started my yelling and ranting at that point about how he got me into this and, if you were in my shoes etc..... But I did not. I knew he was right and instead I began to push.

Finally the baby's head was out and I looked down between my legs and facing me was this little face and neck. The baby looked so peaceful and angelic. I will never forget that moment for as long as I live. The baby's body was still inside of me. Chris looked at the baby and said it looked like a boy face. I knew it was a boy. Chris had been convinced it was a girl. As they suctioned the baby's nose ears etc, the baby, our baby popped its own shoulder out and caught everyone by surprise. My baby knew I was struggling and was trying to help me with this delivery. However I couldn't help but think he had a little push from his special angel. Dr. M announced it's a Boy.

Chris looked at me in shock and said

"Sal it's a boy, it's got balls and everything!"

He was so happy and excited and got to cut the cord and hold the baby. I on the other hand spent the next forty five minutes being stitched while vomiting again. But the moment came when I was able to hold my little boy and Chris and I decided that he would be named Mitchell William. He was a healthy little bundle weighing in at 7lbs 7oz and was 47.5 cm long. They took our baby for testing, cleaning and whatever else and we were moved into the room. We had a private room and Chris asked for a cot and he stayed with me. Mitchell was born at 1:36am on Monday May 22nd 1995. By the time it was all said and done, it was 4:30 am and we were both exhausted.

The staff kept Mitchell in the nursery that night but when the morning came Mitchell needed to be fed. I was trying to give him my breast, but it was not working. He was having a hard time latching on because my nipples were inverted. Chris and I were shocked because we had never had any trouble in the nipple department. But as luck would have it, for some reason, my nipples decided to go the other way and as hard as we tried, we could not get any milk into our little guy. I remember my sister Tina had a few problems breast-feeding and Josie had none. She breastfed all three of her babies and made it look so easy. I thought to myself that if Josie was around, she could give me some guidance, some advice and tell me what worked for her. I guess that was not meant to be. We tried various means throughout my four day stay in the hospital. I know that was a long time but I am thinking it's because they knew about what went down the week before the birth.

The hospital sent a Social Worker to see me. She was lovely and offered her congratulations and her condolences all in the same sentence. She asked if I needed to talk. Of course I needed to talk but that was definitely not the time. We had a pleasant conversation, but I refused any intervention. I didn't need her. I needed to have my sister back. I had just had a baby, a hungry baby and I couldn't give him any of my milk because my nipples for the first time in my life were inverted. That was really my problem and unless the Social Worker could help me with any of that, there was little that she could do for me.

After much frustration and many failed attempts, the nurses suggested that I seriously consider bottle feeding. In all honesty I never had any great longstanding dreams of breastfeeding my baby. I always just assumed I would because really, what could possibly go wrong with these double Ds? I also thought it would be a great way to bond with my baby and save big money too. So the thought of not being able to breastfeed was disappointing, but not earth shattering. So the night my milk came in was the most unpleasant part of the whole lactation ordeal. I had ice packs on my breasts and warm blankets on my whole body. I had a fever all night long. I was afraid to be in hospital by myself and I felt so vulnerable. Chris had only stayed over the first night. So there I was alone. The experience brought back memories of when I was a child and suffered with a lot of fevers. I remembered lying on my bed with my mother by my bedside, putting cold compresses on my forehead and slices of white potatoes. Yes I said potatoes. Apparently the starch from the potato, extracts the heat from the body therefore, lowering the fever. I don't know what it is, but to this day I become frightened when I am sick during the night. I have to admit, that this is one of the time that I miss my mother the most.

After several ice packs and warm microwave blankets, early morning came and my fever was gone. By 3:30 am I had woken up and was no longer afraid or lonely. But I had missed my baby so I walked into the nursery to find him. There he was, my baby Mitchell. I walked over to him and as luck would have it, it was time for his next feeding. The nurses prepared his bottle and he and I snuggled up in the rocking chair. I fed him for the first time with no stress and no fuss. I felt so close to him. I thought to myself, I am a mother now. I have a son and my life will never be the same again. I will never look at life in the same way as I did before. Everything changes when you have a child. A week ago when we buried Josie there were times that I could not see beyond my pain. I wished I had the guts to stop the pain I felt in my heart and the numbness that moved throughout my whole body. But now, I was someone's mother. I had given birth to a life that was growing inside of me just like Josie said I would, and that is truly a miracle. As we rocked back and forth in that chair, I promised my son that I would love him and care for him for the rest of my days. My son was now my Savior.

I have been truly blessed and although Mitchell's birth came at a time when our family faced a tragic loss, he has brought a lot of joy to us all. He is a very special boy who was chosen by the angels, perhaps one special angel. Thank you to Auntie Josie for bringing me my boy. The next day I was discharged and my new life began.

Chapter 37

Life Goes On.....

August 29th, 1995 I wrote:

I've not had a lot of time to put all the thoughts together that are running through my head on paper. Mitchell, my beautiful blue eyed baby boy is sleeping. I am overjoyed with my little boy and know that Nicole will join the family when she is ready to come to us. Mitchell is now three months old, beautiful and healthy. However with every passing month of his life is another month that I have lived my life without Josie. I don't know why I thought that this would get easier. Wishful thinking I suppose. Although I am busier than ever, caring for a new born baby, not a minute or an hour or a day goes by when I don't think of her. I see her face and hear her voice. Sometimes I think I am going to turn around and she will be there. Other times I feel like I am losing my mind. God I miss her so much. Why was she taken from me, her children, all of us? I still have not figured out the

161

reason for all of this.

My brother John called me today from work. He often calls to check up on me and see how the new mommy and baby are doing. He is a sweet guy and an awesome big brother. He told me that he was thinking the other day of a time when Josie was a little girl. He said that she may have been about four years old at the time. She used to sit by the window in the dining room playing where mom used to sit and sew. The fridge was very near and because John was overweight and always in and out of the fridge, he remembers this story. He remembers Josie asking mom why she would see angels every time she looked out the window and up in the sky. At first my mom discarded Josie's claims but Josie insisted that she knew what she saw and that was angels in the sky. Since Josie was never a child to make up stories, mom believed her. Mothers often know that their children are special, so mom said to Josie, that is because you are special and someday you will be an angel too. When I think back, I think that mom always knew that something would happen to Josie. I know I did. John stated that he remembers the story clearly and that he had been meaning to tell me. I suppose it is true that some people are chosen by God and that "only the good people die young" but hell; we want the good people to stick around here as well. As wonderful and comforting as that story of John's was, I still miss her and want her back. I told Johnny how I felt and he agreed. But the whole angel thing is not surprising; Josie was an angel on earth. She did so much for others and never expected anything in return. That is so rare.

When I got off the phone with Johnny, I wondered if I could be half as good a mother as Josie was to her children. I want to be a good person like she was too but dealing with my sister Tina right now is becoming more difficult than ever. Things have gotten worse between us since Josie died. I think what I resent the most is how she has to tell everyone what she is doing for the children. How she is mourning and how stressed out she is. Does she want everyone to feel sorry for her? Well, we all lost a sister. She acts like she is taking the brunt of the pain, the brunt of the responsibility because I am busy with Mitchell. I feel that I am spending a lot of time with the children too. Josie would be appalled. Is it my role to confront her now? I don't know. I have too much anger inside of me. I'm just not sure what to do with it. I am waiting for Josie to give me a sign. I miss talking on the phone with her. She was always a great listener and knew just what to say to calm and support me. She even had a really nice way of putting me in my place too. Oh how I miss having tea with a few cookies and a lot of laughs. Somehow I feel that she will protect us.

I don't know if her spirit is in Mitchell. It's hard to tell especially when you want that to be. She said that she wanted to but I don't know if she had any control over that. She did tell me that she will never leave me. But I don't know, I haven't seen her around anywhere. I told Josie in her last days that it was so hard for me to say good bye to her because I didn't know how I could get on in my life without her. She told me that it was out of our hands. She said to me and I will never forget,

"Sal the book has been written and the path has been laid" I was a little freaked out at this point because Josie doesn't talk this way.

It was almost as though someone was talking through her. Then she said,

"You will be fine, you worry too much"

"How will me and Tina get along without you as our buffer?" I asked.

"We will likely kill each other". She laughed and I laughed too.

"I know Sal, you guys are going to have to get along". She said to me with a smile,

" Do you best." she said. I remember answering.

"I will and I know that Tina will too".

The kids were always Josie's first priority. She told me that if I didn't take care of her kids that she would come and haunt me. That is a bit harsh for someone as sweet as she. But she became serious and told me,

"Be there for Anthony for the finale".

I have made myself available for the kids. They have spent every Friday with me and Mitchell over the summer. John drops them off and goes to work. It has been a wonderful arrangement. They are such great kids and they are a part of her and I hope I will always have them to love. I talk about Josie to them all the time; to the point that, I asked them if it bothered them that I do this. They said no, but I don't know if that is true. They are just kids. Josie asked that we always talk to the kids about her. She wants them to know her through us and not forget her. She also asked that we continue all of the parties and family gatherings. She wants us to have a party for Anthony's upcoming confirmation and Andrea's communion. She wants Andrea to have a scalloped communion dress that she likes. I hope that Tina and I can agree on every-thing during these occasions. She always has a need to take over. Well enough said about that. None of this will bring Josie back.

My life goes on without her and I have a son who unfortunately didn't get to see the person who I am sure would have loved him very much. But he will know everything about her anyways. It is wonderful to see the kids with Mitchell: all three of them. Paul is so involved with Mitchell and comfortable with holding him and feeding him. I know that Josie was always worried about Paul and the fact that he was so intro-verted. She wanted him to express his feelings more often. She saw a lot of herself in Paul. I guess getting close to Mitchell is Josie's way of working through him. Paul said that he will teach Mitchell all there is to know about sports and Anthony and Michael will teach Mitchell how to pick up girls. As for Andrea, she is a wonderful helper. Josie would be proud of her children.

I have been checking on Mitchell. He is so beautiful. He is a wonderful baby. When he sleeps he looks like Chris and when he is awake, he looks like me. It's a win win!

Chapter 38

The Melt Down

On November 17 1995 I wrote:

Basically few of my feelings have changed since the last time I wrote other than the fact that my gorgeous son is almost six months. Other than the fact that he doesn't sleep much, he is a delight. I will probably have more time to write because this week I have started something knew with Mitch. I am putting him down for naps in the am and the pm awake! Yes Awake. He cries a little at first. It kills me but I have to do it otherwise he stays awake all day and that is not good for any of us, especially me. The situation is getting better and I think this knew sleeping arrangement will work.

I just got home from dad's house and I am so furious. I am writing because I have no one to tell this to. Chris is at work, Josie is dead and Tina is a lot like her father. I am over at dad's and we are talking about the fact that one of my niece has a bad cold and somehow this becomes about me and how I almost died when I went to Florida when I was in university and he had to take care of me because of the pneumonia. Well I didn't have pneumonia. I had mononucleosis. He rolled up his eyes in disbelief. God shoot me if I ever do this to my kid. Of course I got very pissed off and told him to think what he wants but that was not what happened. He didn't stop there. He told me that when I was growing up I always thought that I knew everything. I agreed and said that all teenagers are like that but he added that I am still like that. What! I just wanted to grab Mitch my baby and get the hell out of there. But I tried to be patient. After all he was grieving the death of his beloved Josie, mind you we all were. So I tried another approach and explained mononucleosis and how it attacks the body, and the stress of mom dying and school and the house and dealing with him. (I did not say the last part). He minimized everything that I had said. Totally I am so angry. He doesn't realize any of the pain that I went through and all of the sacrifices that I had to make having a sick mother and then no mother at all. When will this ever be resolved? Never that is when. Why is it that all the good people namely Josie had to die and all the bad people in this family are still kicking around. I am so angry with him. Then all of a sudden while he is making sauce for Tina, he asked me how Josie's children are doing and wants me to find out what they need. That is very nice of dad and at the end of the day; he is a very generous man. As for me, I am still feeling angry, frustrated and misunderstood.

I do wish I could talk to Tina about all of this. But I can't talk with her. She is always so stressed and so busy. I wish that she can reduce her stress by going part time. It might be the best thing for her and her family. O God listen to me. Josie, how am I going to continue my life without you? I will never accept this for the rest of my life. Why were you taken away? You were such a beautiful person and you and John built a wonderful family life with great kids. I promise you, your kids will know everything about you. You didn't write anything in your journal about your life before cancer or even about your feelings toward your kids and I am a little angry with you about this. But I guess you know that I will pass on this information on your behalf.

I want to hear your voice again. God it feels like so long ago and then at other times it feels like just yesterday that we were at your house having a tea and a few cookies to satisfy our sweet tooth. Xmas is coming. How will we do it? I suppose the joy that a new baby brings will ease some of my pain. I already bought the kids some nice gifts. I know you wanted to do Andrea's room in floral. So I am giving that to her as a gift; a total room make over and yes, I am replacing the blind! Oh Mitchell's waking up. As usual, it wasn't a long nap.

March 9, 1996 I wrote:

I am really quite disappointed in myself as I haven't taken the opportunities to write as often as I would like or planned to. Then when I do I am so overwhelmed as there is so much to say. Well first is my baby boy Mitchell. He is wonderful, full of life and energy, sometimes too much for me to handle. He will be ten months. He is doing so many things; he is very vocal, has been crawling, standing and moving so fast. He has a very dynamic personality. Always laughing and has a real sense of humor.

I am adjusting to having a baby. My routine is set. I do get bogged down with it and stressed out. Being a stay at home mom has its perks as Josie used to say, but it's not as easy as some of the working mothers may think. I still miss Josie every day. I think I always will but I do have days when I am happy. I know I have to think of his future and I want so much for us to have a happy and good relationship. A child being around a very depressed mother is never a good thing. I am sure it will eventually rub off on the boy. So far he seems happy so I guess I am doing something right. I save my deepest and darkest thoughts for when he is napping which he is finally doing more of thank God or Josie, whoever is responsible. It's hard to believe I have lived without her now for ten months. It seems so long and then at other times it feels like the time has gone by so quickly. It's very confusing. All I have now are memories of her and they are all good. I think she only pissed me off once and she was right anyways. Of course, her children are such wonderful kids and I always look forward to seeing them. I can't wait to tell them so much about their mom when they are ready and wanting to know.

My relationship with dad is always improving. I visit him weekly for an afternoon. He enjoys Mitchell so much. He is so proud and impressed by everything he does. I take dad now to do the groceries and the bank, an outing that he had enjoyed with Josie. I know it and so does he, but we try to make the best of it and move on with life as best we can. Mitchell provides a welcome distraction and brings a lot of joy to dad's life. I think dad respects me more a little now. We still have our disagreements but they are fewer than they used to be.

I know I have to get on with my life. I know what I have to do but it's hard. My heart and my spirit are broken but some days I feel like it's starting to heal. My mind knows what I have to do. I have registered for an interior design course. Grandmamma Louise was kind enough to pay for the course. I really appreciate it. I feel that this will be my next career. I need a fresh start and a new path. I hope I live long enough to fulfill it. If I don't I guess that is the way it was meant to be. I have learned that you can plan out your whole life, but whatever happens, happens. But I still think that it is good to have a plan and set goals. That is what keeps us going. I have a family now and responsibilities so planning for the future is important. I can't lose myself. If I do then I stand to lose everything and every-one that I love, mostly Chris. I know I have to change some of my ways or I fear I will lose him too. I need to really try my best to be happy and sort out all of my feelings. I hope that he will be patient with me a while longer.

April 29th 1996

Well yesterday was our sixth wedding anniver-sary. It was basically uneventful. I had hoped that this year would have been special but it wasn't. I have asked myself, perhaps I am expecting too much. I don't think so. A little sur-prise or a special effort would have been nice. I don't feel like I am special to him or anyone anymore. I feel such sadness right now and I have no one to share it with. I feel very embar-rassed about my feelings. If Josie was here she would be the only person that I would tell. I just can't think of this anymore. It's too painful and sad. Our anniversary is over, Josie is gone and there is nothing that I can do about either.

Chapter 39

A Message From Spirit

On May 14th 1996 I write:

I have had the most amazing experience this morning. Mitch has been waking up at 5:30 in the morning every morning. That is not the amazing part. I do not know why he is up so early. But I am really wearing out fast and feel so tired lately, more than usual. He was finally ready to go back down for his morning nap. I put him in his crib and went into my room to make my bed. Oh it was so tempting. It was like my bed was calling my name and it was hard to resist. I always try to get a few things done while Mitch sleeps, but all I wanted was to nap and so I did. I checked the clock radio and decided I would lie down for about fifteen minutes. It was 8:30 am and I quickly felt myself slipping into a deep comfortable sleep. The next thing I know, I am sitting on a comfortable concrete like bench in the most beautiful garden that I have ever seen. There was golden sunlight everywhere. The sun was so bright yet it did not hurt my eyes. What a beautiful place. I felt very relaxed and at peace when I looked up and couldn't believe who was standing in front of me. It was Josie. I remember gasping in disbelief but so thankful to be seeing her again. She looked so beautiful and healthy just as I had remembered her. Her hair seemed more auburn, but I think that may have been because of the light that was shining around her. I could not take my eyes off of her and I told her that it was so good to see her. I had not seen her in so long. I told her that I was so tired and didn't know what was wrong with me. She smiled at me with a reassuring look that was so familiar to me. Although I did not hear her voice, she told me that I was tired because I was going to have another baby. Another baby? I couldn't believe it. She then told me that she needed to tell me a few things and asked me to walk with her. I do not remember what she told me at that point. But I know that when I woke up, I knew that I was going to be having a baby girl. I was shocked, confused and happy all at the same time. I even felt refreshed as though I had slept the whole morning even though when I opened my eyes, the clock showed 8:35 am. I had only slept for five minutes. I felt that I was with her for so much longer. I did not want my time with her to end. Could this be true? Am I really pregnant again? How could Josie be the messenger of this news on the anniversary of her death? All I know is that seeing her again was incredibly fantastic and the fact that it was my sister delivering the news of my baby girl was even better.

On May 18th 1996 I wrote:

Well what a weekend it has been. Saturday we had a wedding and Josie's one year funeral mass. This is all too familiar. Chris and I had a good time at the wedding, despite the significance of this weekend. Joey stayed with Mitchell. On Sunday, Andrea was crowning Mary at the church so I went to the house to put on her communion dress and get her ready for the mass. She was lovely. I came back home only to have an argument with Chris. He did not get me anything for Mother's day until that afternoon when he ran to the corner store at 4:00pm to get me a card and a frigg'in bunch of flowers. One can only imagine how I felt to say the least. I admit that I have been very depressed and I have also been reliving the experience of Josie's death last year. Not to mention that I already hated Mother's day because I haven't celebrated it since 1981 when my own mother died. But having said all of that, it is the first Mother's day that I am a mother. To top it all off, my period was late so I went in to have a blood test and got my results today at 11:30 am. It was positive and Chris and I will be parents again. I have such mixed emotions. I am very happy because I want another child but I feel very unprepared. I need to make changes again and that is hard for me to do when so much has changed in my life and so quickly. Then I thought of my dream with Josie and the garden and her message telling me that I was pregnant with a baby girl. I really don't know what to make of all of this.

May 30 1996 I wrote:

Well things have been very busy. The day after Victoria Day we had our house painted on the outside. It took all week. In the meantime, Mitchell's first birthday was the same week and his party was on the Sunday May 26th. I decided to do my spring cleaning while I cleaned for this party. I was very excited about it, naturally wanting everything to be perfect. Well the weather was terrible even though it was beautiful the whole week leading up to it. I was disappointed. Most people stayed inside and our home can't really accommodate forty people comfortably or otherwise. Mitchell had loads of fun with all the other kids. The video turned out well and the pictures, we haven't developed yet. Anthony's confirmation was on the Monday. I was so proud of him. He looked so handsome and I know Josie would be proud of him too. Chris was his sponsor. I think Anthony really liked the watch. John's having a barbeque on June 9th. I hope the weather is good. But today and tomorrow I am taking time to relax before we head out to Ottawa. Rico and Erica are getting married on Saturday and then we will have a tour of where daddy was born. Then off to Three Rivers to see Chris' grandmother. I am a little nervous because we have never taken Mitchell on such a long road trip. I hope it will be a safe one.

I have had more time to think about my pregnancy. I feel that because May has been so
hectic, I haven't had much time to think. Chris
and I have talked about the baby. We are both
very happy but it just feels different this time.
There is little time to think and fantasize when
you already have a one year old baby. I don't
really even feel pregnant. I am getting queasy
and I am tired, but other than that, it doesn't
seem like it is real. But today I had a scare when
I peed and wiped. I had a smear of pinkish
discharge. I panicked and then I remembered
talking to Josie about this when I was first
pregnant with Mitchell. She said that the discharge was a sign that I was doing and lifting
too much. That would make sense given everything that I have been doing. I thought, oh my
God, I don't want to lose this baby. I want this
baby very much. I realized that I have been very
unhappy about the timing of this child, not the
child. Okay so now is the big question. I have
a beautiful healthy son, now I want a daughter
too. There are so many things that a mother
and daughter can share. Then again, another
boy would mean a brother for Mitchell and that
would be nice. But if I want to have daughter,
then that would mean a third pregnancy. I don't
necessarily want to stop at two; somehow I like
the idea of three. Josie did it, I probably could
too. Wow I feel like it's been ages since I have
seen her. The last time she came was to confirm
my pregnancy. She was so happy and excited

and I wonder if she will be this baby's spirit. If Josie has any control over on the other side, I know that she will handpick my little girl. She would want that for me and for Andrea too. Her name will be Nicole Josephine.

July 12th 1996 I wrote:

It seems that I have slept the month of June away. I am now in my fourteenth week of pregnancy. The tiredness has been very overwhelming. Basically I try to sleep when Mitchell sleeps and then again earlier in the evening. I seem to be coming out of it as I am up a little later at night. I have gone to two prenatal visits and all seems well. This second pregnancy is really different than my first in many ways. I find myself feeling very queasy but I read somewhere that a lack of rest seems to bring on the nausea more. I think that this is true. It's really difficult to be pregnant when you already have a baby. I am of course much less focused on myself and can't rest when I want to. I remember Josie laughing when I was pregnant with Mitch. She would say "This first pregnancy is your luxury pregnancy, everyone after that isn't so enjoy it". As usual, she was right. This week I spoke with Olwen who just had baby #2- a girl. She said the same thing and her baby is fine. I don't know but I seem worried about this baby. My life is very different now. I don't want any harm to come my baby's way. The reality of the baby seems to be settling in a little more. My waist is getting a little thicker. I am sticking with the same delivery doctor, he was very nice. My due date has been confirmed for January 12 or 13 1997. Somehow I feel our baby is going to come in December 1996. We'll see if my prediction is correct. The kids are all so excited and are already placing their bets on the delivery day. I think Mathew won last time. I have really taken things easy. All I can handle is taking care of Mitchell and light housekeeping. By that I mean barely.

Mitchell is wonderful and is now walking at eleven months. He is active, clever and what a sense of humor. He is charming and charismatic. Really he is everything that I wanted him to be and more. We have the family picnic on Sunday and I am sure that he will have loads of fun with the kids. Last year he had terrible gas and cried most of the time. This year will be different. I am really waiting for my energy to increase in this second trimester. I have things I want and need to do. I have some gifts to make and I want to continue my interior design course and get a few units in before I have the baby. I still have to redo Andrea's room and the new baby's room. So much to do and so little time and energy. For now I will take it easy, but soon, I know that I'll have to plug the motor up my ass and get going! That was one of Josie's favorite lines.

August 20th 1996

Well I am twenty weeks this week and halfway through the pregnancy. There are a lot of things to do. But more importantly my feelings are so different this time. I barely feel pregnant. I've gained only three pounds and it's because I have very little appetite. I go in spurts of hunger. I am not craving anything in particular. My face is a mess with pimples full of water and I barely look pregnant, just fat. I have felt only a few flutters but nothing major as of yet. I look forward to more movement. That is when it will hit me that there is a living being inside of me. Chris and I went for an ultrasound two weeks ago and all was well. The baby measures perfectly and the due date is January13, 1997. I was quite relieved that the baby measured well. I don't know, I keep worrying that something is wrong. To top it all off, I have the flu this weekend and cannot take a thing. I hope Mitchell and Chris don't get what I have. I have an appointment with the doctor on Thursday. Although it was not confirmed 100% because the baby was crouched in fetal position, the technician guessed that it was a girl. Anyways, I know it is a girl because of my dream of Josie and the mysterious box of girly clothes that I found that she left me when I was expecting Mitchell. I will be happy regardless of the baby's gender, but to have a girl this time means our family is complete.

Well I have been keeping very busy lately mostly doing the ceramics. I have almost completed what I have wanted to do for the kids. I am actually getting good at it. I am also making one for Mitchie for xmas and have gotten the kids involved in making their own. Anthony, Paul and

Andrea are enjoying this so much; especially Paul who is so artistic. He is so focused and has an eye for detail just like Josie. Michael and Matthew have even started their own project too. It has been a lot of fun for us all.

I have found a new friend. I have rarely written of her and I am not sure why. She is Jennifer and she lives across the street. She is a very nice person and we have become quite close. We have a lot in common and we have done a lot of things together. We have made strawberry and raspberries jam, waffles and are doing ceramics too. It's really nice to have her as a neighbor. We look out our living room windows to see if the other is out on the porch. We have had some really long talks too and we seem to understand each other. It's nice to have that again. She has certainly not replaced Josie, but it is nice to report the daily events to someone again. Unfortunately they are renters and the day will come when they will move. I worry about that but I know that is selfish. Grand-mama Louise came on Thursday evening and left Friday afternoon. It was a short visit, she came with her sister Odette. It was nice to see Odette. They are excited about the new baby and Aunt Odette and Mitchell got along really well. He just loved her.

I just found out last week from Angie that she had a dream about Josie. Apparently she told Angie that it was not an easy thing for her to come and see her. She said that she had to do

a lot in order to come but said this was important. She asked Angie to do her a favor and tell
her sisters to stop their bitching. She added
that we are bitching about stupid things. She
also told Angie that she wants everyone to be
close and then she left. I have mixed feelings
about this and I know that this information was
difficult to pass along. I suppose that Josie sees
things from a different perspective from where
ever she is and sees our bickering as futile. I
don't know. Such is my life now. I have to go.
I am so tired and the cold is getting more con-
gested. Goodnite.

On August 23rd 1996 I wrote:

Oh my God. Call me crazy but the strangest
thing happened last night. I went to an Interiors
class on faux finishing and I was so sick with
this cold. I probably shouldn't have even gone.
I was coughing all night. Anyways, Chris was
caring for Mitchell and by the time I got home,
he had already put the baby to bed. I check my
son every night before I close my eyes, but last
night I did not and instead I went right to bed. I
was so sick and I knew that if Mitchell woke up
through the night that I would have to be the one
to care for him. As great of a father as Chris is,
no one can wake him when he is in deep sleep.
It is almost grounds for a divorce. So I prayed
to whomever to let my baby sleep through the
night so that I could sleep too. Morning came
and I realized that I had not gotten up in the
night to tend to the baby. But I did remember a

dream that I had in the night that Mitchell was being rocked in his rocking chair by none other than his auntie Josie. I remembered this so well. He was cradled in her arms and she was staring at him and rocking him back to sleep. It felt so real. But how real could this be? I jumped out of bed and ran into Mitchell's room and there he lay, still asleep with the same little pajama sleeper that I saw him in when he was being rocked by Josie. I ran back into my room and woke Chris up. He had to get up anyways and I asked him if he got up with Mitchell or if I did check on him before I went to bed. He answered no to both questions. I sat there on my bed not knowing what to make of all of this. If I did not check my baby before I went to bed then how would I know which pajama sleeper he was wearing when he was being cradled by Josie? Is this just a coincidence or did something really special happen last night? Could it be that Josie is around us like she said she would? I guess she is helping me after all.

August 28 1996 I wrote:

Good morning. Mitchie is already asleep for his morning nap and it is 9:30 am. That is because he is still getting up at 5:30 am every morning. I couldn't stay up with him so Chris did. I could not move. But this morning I noticed a new tooth. Not his eye tooth but the one behind it. He is doing fine but is much testier now. He understands the word no and often ignores it. This is getting more difficult. The pregnancy is going well and I felt the baby thumping from the outside. At other times I feel gentle pitter patters. I'm still not gaining weight. I have very little appetite and I am concerned about the baby getting the proper nutrients. I have just gotten over the flu so that didn't help either.

So much else has happened this past week. Chris has gotten a new position within the company. It's what he has wanted for a long time. It's called an AC position. He is very happy and I am happy for him but it will take him away a lot.

October 18, 1996 I wrote:

I just can't seem to keep up. I had a second ultrasound on October 16th because my placenta was a bit low and they needed to check if it moved up. Basically it has and the placenta is in the proper position and baby is fine. Baby is also a girl. It was confirmed and although I figured it would be, I was still stunned and overjoyed!! I can't believe I will have the opportunity of having that mother daughter relationship that I have longed for my whole life. I feel truly blessed that I already have a wonderful little boy and now a girl. When the technician confirmed it, the first thing I said to myself was 'Thank you Josie". I know that she was instrumental. She always wanted me to have a daughter. Andrea was so happy and so was dad. Tina and my sister in law, Doris on the other hand are still quite skeptical. They will believe it when they see the baby. After all, they didn't have a girl why should I! Tina has two great sons and having a third baby would have been too risky. I know that she would have loved to have a daughter too. We have been getting along fine lately but the other day we were talking about Nicole's baptism and it didn't end well. I thought she was assuming things, she thought I was over-reacting. All these thoughts in my head. She makes me crazy. I can't talk about this anymore. None of this will bring Josie back.

I am twenty eight weeks and I've gained 4lbs thus far. Unbelievable, Mitchie and I are having wonderful days. I love him so much. I feel sad because soon he will have to share his mommy. I wonder if he knows or understands this. He has a lovely personality but a temperamental streak too. I suppose he is building character. I am still keeping very busy. Whoever said that staying at home was easy was very wrong. I wish I had Josie to spend time with. Seventeen months ago today, was her funeral. God how I still miss her. I think I always will. I still don't understand and I want her back. It is comforting to know that both of my children have a special guardian angel and that is their Auntie Josie.

Chapter 40

Some Things Just Can't Be Explained!

November 9/96 I wrote:

The weeks are going by quicker and it is only a matter of time before our new baby girl is born. Chris has been really busy at work and traveling a lot more with this new position. I feel very alone. The other night I put Mitchell down to sleep and John and I talked on the phone for hours about Josie. We talked about how much we loved her and how much we miss her now. Anthony, Paul and Andrea were asleep too. We are sure that Josie is watching over them all the time. John is managing through the strength that he feels is given to him by Josie. He admits that she made life look so easy but he is doing his best with the children. He hopes that she would approve. I assured him that she would approve and that he is not alone. The family is there to help and support him and the children. They feel our love but we know that they are missing their mother. John and I talk regularly and there are many times when words can't describe our pain so we both just cry and cry. That is what happened to us the other night. Only something extraordinary happened while I was crying on the phone with John. We were talking about how lost we felt without her in our lives when I started to cry. I was sitting at the dining room table wiping my tears with my bare hands, when all of a sudden, I opened my eyes to get up and grab a tissue, when there lying on the table was a clean, unused tissue. I looked around the room and did not see any tissues nearby. I knew that I had not plucked this tissue from a box, yet it was lying right beside my right hand. How did this tissue get there? I suddenly stopped crying and as embarrassed as I was, I told John about what had just happened. We were both very quiet and agreed that in some strange way Josie is still around us taking care of us and giving us comfort.

December 30, 1996 I wrote:

I had an appointment with the doctor today. When he examined me, he told me that the baby was no longer in a head down position. She had moved and was now feet first. I told the doctor that last Thursday I felt a real tumble. It felt like the baby was doing somersaults in my belly and my whole world was upside down. I remember that I felt dizzy and had to sit down and have some water. I also felt some pain but it passed. I remember feeling scared and Chris and I were unsure what to do. Before long, I was starting to feel settled and went to bed. Now this I thought. The doctor told me that he had to manipulate the baby back to the head down position. Oh my God that was so painful. I was in tears as he pulled and stretched and pushed on my belly. The important thing is that he was successful. He gave me an internal and baby girl was back in position. Her heartbeat was still at 140 and everything was fine. He is concerned that the baby may turn again and that she will be breech. I felt so panicked but I didn't want to show that so I acted calm, otherwise he wouldn't tell me anything. Basically he said that for the baby to have moved at this stage, means that she has a lot of room to move in there which may indicate that she is small. Well that was it. I have caused this because of my poor appetite and I have not been eating enough or many of the healthy foods that I did the first time. He wants to book me in on Monday January 6th for an ultrasound at 2:00 pm to determine whether the baby has moved positions and to see how big she is. I am worried for my baby girl-Nicole. Vaginal delivery was no picnic. I had stitches all the way up my ass, but at least no one could see those scars. I don't want a c-section but if that is the safest way to get my baby out then that is what will be done. As I have been writing, she has not stopped moving. She is a real mover and a shaker. Although I was initially devastated by this news, I have thought things through. I believe that all will be well. But I will feel much better after the ultrasound on Monday. I pray everything is fine and that he doesn't see the need to admit me because Chris has to go away for a presentation. He says he can't get out of it. He actually spoke with the director, but has to go. He is very afraid that I will deliver while he is away. I hope that doesn't happen. Chris was so involved in Mitchell's birth; I know he would be devastated if he missed this one.

Everything is ready, room, clothes, car seat etc. The bags are packed and I am now in low gear, resting in the evenings and napping by day with Mitchell. I think it's time that I need right now. I have a very difficult year ahead of me. I know I need at least a few weeks of peace and rest.

January 4 1997 I wrote:

Preparing for Christmas was much more of a struggle than I thought. I made a lot of gifts from ceramics and that took a lot of time and energy. I also made a lot of ornaments for the tree. This is my attempt to start some family traditions for our children when we are gone. This was the first Christmas spent with Chris' mom. She joined us on the eve at Tina's house and that was very nice. On Christmas day we stayed home and had dinner with Louise and daddy came over for the day. Christmas will never really be the same without Josie. She is gone. Why am I still in so much shock? It's funny though, I have been feeling her so near lately. Mitchell added a new little spark to the holidays. It was really his first Christmas where he was able to open presents and have fun. Brother John dressed as Santa. He always makes a great Santa. Andrew and Mitchell's little faces were just in awe. It was wonderful. All the children had a great time. Chris' job is going well and he is happy and stressed as a result. Our relationship has improved, although I wonder if we will ever have sex again. We stopped at eight months. I just couldn't move anymore. To date I have now gained seventeen pounds. Mitchie is now 19 months and is so delightful and defiant too. He is really developing his personality and his vocabulary is amazing. I am really not sure that he understands that another little person, a female to boot, is about to enter his world. Some days I am not sure if I am ready for two babies under two. But we are now one week away from the due date. I can only hope for the best at this point and pray and believe that our special angel up there will protect us. As I have always said, Josie has always been there for me and she has never let me down. My life will be forever changed. Again.

Chapter 41

Welcome Nicole Josephine

January 24, 1997 I wrote:

Well needless to say, I have been quite busy since having Nicole. Yes we had our baby girl and now we have one of each. I had quite the scare when at thirty- eight weeks; Nicole decided to flip to a breech position. It was a very painful experience when Dr. M manipulated my stomach in order to move the baby out of the breech and in a head down position. Dr. M was concerned that the baby was too small because she had a lot of room to move around. He quickly booked me in for an ultrasound and a quick visit with him on the 30th. I was still worried because a few days after the manual manipulation, I felt her move again like she had before when she moved to a breach position. I was mentally preparing myself for a c-section all the while wondering if my poor diet and lack of proper sleep was contributing to what was happening. I was very afraid and wondering if my baby was going to be okay. The night before my ultrasound, I felt her moving big time and it caused me a lot of pain in my abdomen. She had beared down low in head down position and I knew it. My prayers had been answered. When I went to the appointment the next day, the ultrasound technician told me that the baby was head down and that all was normal. She estimated that the baby weighed about 7lbs 6oz, seemed healthy and had lots of hair. She did not give me a picture because the baby's face was facing my back. She said that she was unable to confirm the sex of the baby because of the position as well. But that was fine. I knew she was a girl anyways. Following my ultrasound, I went to see Dr. M who confirmed that the baby was healthy and told me that sometimes things cannot be explained. He decided that he wanted me to be booked for an induction; no not to the hall of fame, but to the hospital as he was fearful that the baby may move again. He did not want to take any chances. I was in full agreement but then picking out a date was difficult. Chris was away on business and would not be home until late in the evening on Tuesday. Joey was watching Mitchell for me and was going to stay the night so that I would not be alone. Joey is more than a nephew; he is the little brother I never had. He is so sweet and really cares about us. So all in all, Tuesday was out of the question. So that left Wednesday the 8th.

That sounded good as that is Elvis Presley's birthday and Joey's birthday too. It didn't matter because that day was all booked anyways. So Thursday January 9th was the day. It was open and available and I was booked that day to have my baby girl-Nicole. The day before on the Wednesday, at about 9:00 am my mucus plug broke and I was unsure as to what was going to happen next. I stayed calm and slowly went about my business doing the laundry and some light cleaning before reporting to the hospital. Surprisingly I slept the night and got the call at 7:30 am from the hospital. They were ready for me. Wow I suddenly became nervous and quickly phoned Joey who was on standby to come over and stay with Mitchell. Then I called everyone else to tell them that we were on our way. It broke my heart to leave Mitchie knowing that I wouldn't see him for a couple of days. Joey arrived quickly and Chris and I were off to the hospital. I was hooked up to the intravenous and received the induction medication at about 10:30 am and by 1:00 pm I was in hard contractions. I sustained the pain until about 3:00pm and then I asked for the epidural. What is it with me and 3:00pm? If I remember correctly that was my limit when I delivered Mitchell as well. By 3:30pm I had received the epidural. I didn't get a spinal one because of the itching. It went through my intravenous and I only felt a mild itch. This time I was awake. Wide awake and I waited and waited. They kept checking me and I was 2-3 cm dilated then I was 4 cm dilated. But then by the dinner hour I was 8cm and at 6:30pm Dr. M came in to break my water. From that point on, I was experiencing something that I never had the first time. It was a real bearing down feeling. I felt the baby was really pushing down low. To the point that if I coughed or sneezed, she would have come out. By 7:15 pm the nursing staff was changing and Joanne came to introduce herself. She was lovely as all the nurses were but at this point I was not interested in small talk. I quickly gave Joanne a rundown of what had been going on and told her that I felt it was time. She didn't really take me too seriously which was really starting to piss me off. She told me that according to the chart, I was only 8 cm forty five minutes ago. I kind of chuckled with a nervous but frustrated laugh and explained to her what I was feeling. She was still stalling until I finally took a hard stand. When I do that I usually start my sentences with what else but Listen....check me for yourself or get the doctor because this baby wants out!!! By this point it was 7:30 and she took me seriously and checked me only to leave the room in a complete panic calling for the doctor. Other nursing staff came rushing in with Dr. M and I hear her say that the baby's head was right there. Things were moving at this point and they were all racing about getting the tray and all the other equipment ready. They were not prepared because they thought that I had about another few hours yet. While everyone was scurrying about, all I wanted to do was push but it seemed that no one was paying any attention to me. So I call out a "Hello I need to push" and Dr.

M got into position. He said "Four good pushes and this baby will be out". He was right and since I was awake and doing fairly well, I asked for the mirror and saw everything. In four or five pushes she was out and I saw her whole little body come out of mine. Dr. M. announced "It's a girl". Chris and I were so happy. She scored a 9 out of 10 on the apgar test and was perfect. I had been so worried. Nicole Josephine was born on Thursday January 9th 1997 at 7:57 pm. Chris held her first while I was being cleaned and stitched-only five stitches this time. I couldn't believe it. Then I got to hold her. I felt quite emotional. In my arms was my beautiful daughter and my dream had come true. We moved on up to the room and then my pain started. To make a long story short, I swelled up on one side of my labia. It was protruding and was very painful. After several ice packs and zits baths, I got rid of it but it took three weeks. Apparently this happens when you have a quick delivery. I came home on Saturday morning. Nicole Josephine had no jaundice and has been gaining weight rapidly.

Chapter 42

The Million Dollar Family

February 12, 1997 I wrote:

Nicole is a perfect baby. She is a good- natured baby. She is just over a month now and I have yet to spend the whole night awake with her. She has been eating and sleeping. Already she is up to five ounces of milk. She is having more awake time now which is great and she can look at you now when you talk to her. Mitchie is quite affectionate toward her and wants to kiss her and hug her, but then turns around and slaps her or squeezes her. He loves her hair because it is so soft. He rubs his lips on her hair and giggles because it tickles. Then he pulls it. He is just a baby himself. He will be twenty-one months next week. I am hanging in. I am busy but not frantic. I am tired but not yet exhausted. The only thing that is wearing me down is Mitchie's behavior these past few weeks. I am not sure it's the eye teeth breaking through or the terrible twos or even Nicole's arrival. I am sure it is a little bit of everything. He is whipping things around and crying a lot. I am about to lose it with him. I am trying to be patient but all I feel like doing is yelling and I don't want to be that way. I am sure that it can't be easy adjusting to another little person around who is taking up a lot of my time and attention. He has to share me now and I suppose he is letting me know that he doesn't like it. I need to find a solution and I need to be more patient. Otherwise I have been doing well. At three weeks, Chris and I had resumed. Yes once I got rid of that thing on my labia, we were able to start having sex again and it's been great. We have shared a real closeness. I feel really free and in love with my husband. He has been feeling great which really makes all the difference. Feeling connected to him in that way makes me feel fantastic. We are both so happy with our new family and seem to agree that we will not plan for a third child. Okay it's mostly me. If I wanted to Chris would support it but I don't feel that it's in the cards. We have two beautiful healthy children, one of each sex and I just want to concentrate on them. They are nineteen months apart which has sent my body over the edge and I would have to wait a couple of years to have the third. I will soon be 35 this year. I'm too old and I don't think that I would be able to handle three kids. Chris understands this but he does not want me to have the operation. He feels that I have been through enough just having the babies. He suggested that he have a vasectomy in the near future. Wow that meant a lot to me.

Chris is so patient and understanding with the children. He spends a lot of time with Mitchell, playing with him. As for Nicole, he has really developed a bond with her; even sooner than I did. She melts in his arms and sleeps on his chest a lot. She doesn't do that with me. I think it's the boobs. Anyways I love them both and will devote my life to raising them into healthy adults. I realize that I have goals too. There are things that I want to do in my life for me. Oh I hear the babies. I must go now.

February 14,1997 I wrote:

Well it's another Valentine day gone down the drain. Only this time it started off great. Chris and I have been getting along really well. We have been communicating, hardly arguing at all and our love making has been absolutely fantastic. I've been really happy with our relationship and feel like we have been on the right track. This past week has been demanding at work for Chris and therefore he has been preoccupied. Last night he was preparing for a presentation for this morning and I asked him if he felt we were drifting apart. He said that he felt we were not and explained that he was preoccupied with the presentation. He also told me that he was looking forward to tonight. I told him that I felt nervous about Valentine's Day and he hugged me and assured me that he was not going to forget and it would be a wonderful evening. I believed him and he sounded sincere and then I went to bed.

This afternoon I received beautiful roses pink ones, my favorite and one red one because it is Valentine's Day. I was really happy and I thought, he didn't forget and made the effort. I thought to myself, "Things are looking up". So this afternoon I am running around with the babies, getting myself all ready and making a nice dinner. Chris gets home from work and during the get the dinner on the table rush, he hands me this card. My hands were full, I was trying to get everything on the table at the same time and I didn't feel that this was the right time to open a card. So I told this to Chris in a tone that he did not feel was nice. Basically I said "Not now, later" and he became so angry with me that he walked away. Since we were on the topic of cards, his mother sent him one so I passed that along to him. He told me that he was so upset that he could not read it. When I asked him why he stated that he was so upset that I did not take his card and when I explained that it was a chaotic moment, he stated that he was trying to break that moment. He was really angry with me and I couldn't believe it. I stood there not knowing what to say or do. This was ridiculous. For me, the evening was not the same. I too had a card for him and one that Mitchie had made. I thought in my mind we would exchange cards after dinner. I am so upset and disappointed.

I thought to myself, "Why can't we have a Valentine's Day that is without argument or miscommunication?

I walked over to the stove, shut everything off and told him to have dinner with himself and went downstairs in the basement. I have been down here ever since. Mitchie was crying for me and asking for me and Nicole has been crying too. Chris came downstairs at one point and told me that he doesn't want things to be this way. Well neither do I. He always has a way of messing things up. He wants to have dinner as a family and wants to forget about what happened and carry on. I wish I could, but I can't. This is obviously a problem that I have. I can't seem to do that. My heart doesn't feel the same when shit like this happens. Why can't I? My life would be so much easier if I could. Chris has always had a problem with doing and saying the right thing. Well today he did it half right. He remembered to order me the flowers but then screws up and gives me this card on the fly. I was willing to overlook that but then, he gets mad at me for my reaction and now I am downstairs in the basement on Valentine's Day alone and he is upstairs with the kids. Josie would probably tell me that I am over-reacting and tell me to get my ass on upstairs. But how can I go back upstairs and make nice and pretend that everything is fine. I just can't do that. I think I will stay down here and clean the basement or something. Why does life, my life have to be this way. Why do things happen smoothly for others but not for me? Why did something so stupid have to end up like this? I feel crushed and hurt. I was looking so forward to tonight and now it is gone. I don't know how to change my feelings that are in my heart. I want to stay down here to hurt him like he hurt me. But I am hurting my son who keeps on asking for me. I can hear him and I feel like a terrible mother now. I guess I am. I don't know what to do. I know that I have so much to be grateful for but I also know that I am stuck in this terrible place of sadness and loneliness.

February 21 1997 I wrote:

Well, I went back upstairs after two hours of being downstairs in the basement. I was frozen to the bone. We ended up salvaging the evening and all in all it ended up fine. Needless to say, I still feel the event was tarnished again this year. We decided that I need to change this type of attitude and to avoid any further messes, we are going to plan what we want to do ahead of time on such events like anniversary, birthdays etc. We spent much of this week talking about how we or I need to change. We have made a commitment that we want to be together because we are in love and want to raise our children together. We want the next years together to be different and better. I have made contact with my angels as a result, things seem brighter. I know what I need to do to get started. I have a separate book that I have started for these writings. I think I will write now because I feel like a terrible mother today. I have done nothing but yell at Mitchell. He and Nicole are asleep. I think I am just tired. It was a hard day yesterday. Nicole did not sleep at all and that is unusual for her. She needed to be hugged and cuddled all day so I carried her around everywhere which I am sure brought out a lot of jealousy in Mitchell. As a result, he has been acting out. Voila! I need some help. I think I need someone to talk to. Gone are the days of tea and cookies. I feel so alone.

Chapter 43

Alone Again

February 25, 1997 I wrote:

Chris has been in North Carolina for a couple of days and he arrives home tomorrow night on his birthday. I bought him a really nice watch and Mitchie and I will make him a card. I miss him but I am managing fine. Tonight I watched this child abduction movie and I am terrified. I knew that I should not have watched it but I could not turn it off. The kids have been great but it's hard raising two babies especially when I am alone. Chris will be away a lot in the upcoming months. I am sure that I will manage fine. All this will seem more worth it when he starts making more money. Nicole is seven weeks old. I feel like she has always been around. She is a wonderful baby and is growing so fast. I really love her already.

March 12, 1997 I wrote:

I took Nicole to see the doctor yesterday. She weighs 12lbs 6oz at only two months. She is growing so quickly. She is a delight and is smiling a lot now. She is recognizing our voices now and Mitchie is getting a real kick out of her. He is really good with her but the odd time, gives her a little extra kick. He doesn't know it yet, but he will get a rude awakening when she starts the biting stage.

Chris has been in Chicago this week and off to Georgia next week. It has been a really difficult month because I have been all alone with the kids. They have been great but there are very few breaks. I have not heard from Chris this week because I asked him not to call me. We have really been struggling and I don't know where we are headed. We have done nothing but argue. I love him so much but I feel that so much has changed between us. Sure there is more pressure, more responsibilities; we have kids and a house. Although things have changed, much of our conflict issues are still the same. I feel that we go around and around in circles. I am hoping that by not talking this week, it will help us to realize what we have and how we feel about each other. I hope he has done some thinking about our life together and our future. He comes home on Friday night and I am nervous to see him. What will he tell me? I am probably expecting too much, thinking that he would do some thinking himself. After all, he is a guy. It's Thursday night and he still has not phoned me. I thought he would have by now even though I told him not to. I am not sure why if it's because he is doing what I asked or if it is because he is still angry with me. I miss him and want to forget everything that happened before he left and give him a big kiss and a hug when he comes home and make love all night. Once the kids are in bed of course! Should I remain distant and go back and try to resolve what happened? I know that whatever happens when he walks through that door will set the tone for the rest of the weekend. I know that all too well, but I do not know which way to go. I am very confused. I don't have anyone that I can talk to about this. Maybe I should take this up with my angels. I haven't written to them as I had planned. Maybe they can help. I think that is what I will do. I need their help right now.

August 11, 1997 I wrote:

I have taken up with my angel writing and have neglected my journal. Certainly since March, my life has taken a turn for the better. Chris is no longer traveling. He switched to another department. The pressure was too much for a young family. He missed us and we missed him. I missed him and his companionship, help and support. I do not feel as alone as I did before. It has really made me appreciate him more. Our relationship has really improved and we are both happy about that. The children are thrilled. Nicole is now in her seventh month and is growing beautifully. She is a lovely baby and I will miss this baby stage with her as she grows older. Maybe because I know that she will be my last baby. I know that through my experience with Mitchie, that there are more good times ahead. She is wanting to explore and the two of them have gotten into a few scrapes already. They are both so beautiful and I feel so blessed to have them in my life. Life is getting a little easier with the kids. Mitchie is now in his 27th month and has a full vocabulary already. He is so bright, very affectionate and sensitive. He has however inherited my quick temper but you've got to take the good with the bad. The two of them are interacting well and I am so happy about that. We are unfortunately going through the "mine" stage which creates some problems between them, but Nicole is holding her own.

On some days, I am still missing Josie as much as I did since the first day she died. I am still trying to figure out how I can fill that void and that longing for her. Yesterday we celebrated Paul's 13th birthday. He is such a beautiful boy. The celebration was a little late due to them being on vacation. Every time I go there it is so difficult because I feel her absence so much. Everything in that house has a memory. All of the things we shopped for, and all the other things that meant a lot to her. We spent so much time there together. We enjoyed so many cups of tea in that house and when I left dad's and moved into my own apartment, her house became my home. My roots; a place I could always go back to and now its not the same, because she is not there. You know, even this journal was bought with Josie in mind. After her diagnosis, she was told that keeping a journal would be a helpful way to release a lot of her feelings. Josie's journal was hardly begun because her life had ended so quickly. In mine, there are so many painful feelings of grief written in the pages of this journal. I hope that the next one I start will be the beginning of more happier and joyful times!

Chapter 44

My Dearest Angels

AT AN early age, I found myself challenging many of the teachings that I had received at school and from my parents. I really wanted to believe much of what I had learned my whole life. But I was stuck on the idea that if God was so good then why would he let all the good people die? I had asked that question so many times in the five years that mom was sick and dying. If God was good, then why would he allow my mother to suffer in this way? I was fortunate that I was able to turn to the chaplain and my religion teacher at the high school where I attended. They helped me to make some sense of it all. But I was still left with a lot of unanswered questions. Sometimes you just have to accept things without knowing why.

At that time in my life, I had decided that I was never going to accept what happened to our mother and to me. Instead, I learned to live without her in my life and for a while, I was doing a great job. Once I got passed the numbness, I started to busy myself to the point that I rarely allowed any time to think about my mother, let alone shed any more tears for her. I kept going for several years at that pace until I was depleted of all my energy. I felt like I had a flu that never went away, so I decided to pay a visit to Dr. R for some blood tests. One look at me and he asked me,

"What are you running from"?

By asking me that one question, he opened up a fountain of tears. I had been running from my pain; a pain that left me feeling alone, abandoned and unloved. One week later, I went back to see the doctor. My test results were in and revealed that I had a severe case of mononucleosis. He explained that this virus had attacked my immune system and that is why I was so sick and fatigued. I spent the next year recuperating and gaining more of my strength as I completed my fourth year in University.

I continued to live my life as a motherless daughter and was actually learning to live without her. Then, fourteen years later, cancer came barging into our lives again when Josie got diagnosed. We were all asking ourselves why. Why her? Why so young? Why? Why? Why? My search to answer "Why" continued, as I withdrew deeper. I found myself alone in my depression feeling like no one could understand; not even Chris, whom I shared a life with full of promise and excitement. I knew that our relationship had been affected. I knew that I had lost a part of myself and I did not know how to get it back. Would I ever be the person that I was before Josie died? I was not so sure. I think that person is gone and I had to discover who I was now. The question was, how was I going to do that? I have always believed in the power of therapy and the benefit of reaching out to someone in the helping profession. But I had two babies, a husband who traveled for work, and no one to care for my children so that I could go for the counseling that I knew I needed. I had friends but they had busy lives too. So I decided that I needed to help myself.

I had been keeping a journal since the year prior to Josie's death. I found it to be a helpful way to get clarity and provide

me a safe outlet to express myself and my feelings. In the
years after Josie died, I had learned about Angel Writing. I
can honestly say that I am unsure how I first learned about
this. Whether it was through one of the books I had been
reading or The Oprah Show, I had decided that I would
learn more about this special communication. And that is
what I did. I came across several books and started to read
and learn about Angel writing. One book called Angelspeake,
describes Angel writing as:

"An energy that comes directly from God; a vibratory
energy. Angels carry out God's plan and can be a support
to those who need it. Through writing to your angels, you
connect your spiritual and physical self."2

That information was enough to peak my interest. But
I was cautious as I did not want to get into anything really
weird. Yet I had a strong feeling that this would be an outlet to
express my feelings. So I read on. It seemed simple as I had
to first ask about something specific that was on my mind. I
thought that would be easy because I had a lot of questions
and all I could think about was what I had lost. I had to allow
it to happen by quieting my mind and receive the messages
that were being communicated to me by the angels. I thought
that part would probably be the most difficult because I had
never really done anything like this before. Of course the last
step was gratitude. Thanking them for coming and offering
their guidance. In some ways it all felt strange, but in many
others ways, it sounded like exactly what I needed.

I was eager to start this new communication and had gotten
myself a new writing book especially for this occasion. For a
while I needed to practice and I felt that I was getting the hang
of it. There were times that I felt their responses were really
me since I was holding the pen. But as each day passed, I

2 Barbara Mark and Trudy Griswold, Angelspeake; A guide how to talk with your
angels: (New York: Simon & Schuster 1995)

continued to meet with my angels and realized that my hand and my mind were being guided by something that I could not see or touch, but yet I knew was present. I suppose this was what they meant when they said connecting your spiritual and physical self. I would often begin this ritual by closing my eyes and taking a few deep breaths, just enough to relax me and clear my thoughts; a quick prayer to ask for guidance and then I would start writing. The following is an example of one of the many Angel Writings that I have written.

On March 26th 1997 I wrote

My Dearest Angels

The children are both down for their afternoon nap and I am upstairs in the attic. It was not easy to get their naps to co-ordinate, but I am glad that I will have a few hours to myself. I must call dad as I always do at this time, but I really wanted to write to you first. I wanted to thank you for your messages over the past few days. I have taken your advice and have noticed that Christopher and I seem so much happier. We had such a wonderful night and we talked and laughed. I didn't want it to end. Angels, will our happiness with one another continue? I feel so alone and unhappy most of the time. I am still missing Josie so much. I know that my relationship with Tina is improving slowly but I wish I could talk with her more. I don't want to feel like this anymore. Please give me some guidance and direction. I am searching for happiness in my life and in my marriage.

My Dearest Salvina, we are pleased that you are happy. You deserve happiness and have been without for a long time. Look to those who can help you with the children. Your sister Tina is there for you. Your children enjoy their time with her and her boys. Tina is changing slowly. You have a great impact on her and she values what you think. You are a significant person in her life. She needs you and you will be there for her to give her perspective on life. You need her too in a different way. She is the source of your family now and you have fought that in the past, but are slowly accepting that as a good thing. Take every opportunity to spend time with Christopher away from your home. He loves you very much but misses the fun loving woman that he fell in love with. Salvina, your pain is still very strong. You will always love your sister Josie. Your sorrow for Josie is deep. She is with you always and with your children too. Her death was destined. She was placed in your life to teach you many things. You didn't know at the time how much you were learning from her, but you are slowly seeing it now. Josie loved you very much and you are one of the key people aside from her husband and children, that she had difficulty leaving behind. You brought much to her life, more than you think. You must treasure these memories of her and remember that her spirit is within you all the time. Your pain will lessen Salvina, but don't be afraid of forgetting her, for you never will. She is helping Chris also. She loved him too and wants him to succeed for him but also for you. You must focus on your life with your husband and children and the happiness within yourself. We have said much

today. Go and do other things. All will be fine.
You need to believe and all will be provided.

Thank you angels for all of your insight and
guidance. I will do my best to live a better life
and I am committed to allowing happiness in
my life and peace within myself.

My Angel writings often gave me hope and took away my
fear and loneliness. My Angels became my trusted friends;
someone that was always there for me whenever I needed
them, like Josie. There were times when the words were
coming so quickly that I was scrambling to get them on the
pages. Oftentimes, I had forgotten what I had written because
I was in a trance while I was receiving these messages. I
realize now as I reflect on this experience that my Angel
writings were my therapy and through these writings I was
encouraged to take the steps that would move me forward in
my life. In many ways, I feel that their guidance helped me
become a better mother, helped me find value in my marriage and overall gave me the strength to fight through my
grief and achieve the happiness that I realized I deserved.

Chapter 45

New Beginnings

I LOVED OUR home. It was a solid 1930 all brick house with original wood trim, pocket doors and leaded crystal glass windows. And of course, hardwood floors throughout. There was no grand staircase, I would have loved that, but instead, we had a beautiful wood burning fireplace in the living room. It was a two story house with a third floor walk up attic. It ended up being my favorite place in the whole house. It was just the two of us when we bought the home in the spring of 1993. We knew that this would be the home where we would start our family.

But first things first, we had to paint. I remember feeling so excited as we both had many ideas for each of the rooms. We went right to it and had every room in the house painted within the first two weeks. A paint brush in my hand, and Chris as my clean- up crew, we completed the look. It was a comfortable home with a touch of glam. Chris and I were thrilled to host Christmas Eve that year with the family. It was the first of many we thought, but I was so nervous to have everyone there. I was a wreck. Everything had to be perfect and I remember trying out all of these new recipes. In my mind that was the only way to avoid comparison of any of my sister's recipes. It is tough being the little sister. Especially when you have one sister who is an excellent cook and another who could have been a professional baker, had she lived long enough to pursue her talent. I acknowledge that I am neither. So my focus was to ensure that everything looked fabulous and I have gotten really good at paying attention to those details. If anyone complained that nothing tasted right, at least they could say that everything looked nice! My sisters and their families, along with dad were so complimentary and it meant so much to us both but especially to me. Their approval meant that I did well. We had backyard parties too with the family and our friends. I remember such good times in the backyard. We had a lovely yard with jasmine trees, purple iris, orange tiger lilies, ferns, lilies of the valley and a big beautiful snowball tree that covered this cute little dog house. I ended up painting it and added some finishing touches with my block painting kit. We never had a dog but it became a cozy spot for our two black and white cats at the time, Sherlock and Watson.

Chris and I lived there for two years before we brought our first baby home in 1995 and then our second in 1997. So much had already changed in our lives and so unexpectedly. We ended up living in that house for seven years. I had gone back to work after being away from the workforce for five years and we started thinking about the schools in the neighborhood. It is so true how when you have children, you think about these things. There were other reasons for wanting to move. We needed a bigger space for our growing family and a fresh start. I started to feel like I needed a change which is so unlike me. I usually fight change every step of the way. But this time, I knew that it needed to happen. We had some wonderful times in our home, but I needed to be honest with myself. I shed a lot of tears in that house too. It had become a place where I associated with pain, suffering and loneliness.

My longing for Josie was so deep during the time I lived in that home. My emotions were so raw and I remember escaping to the attic when the babies were down for their afternoon nap. I would write to my angels and pour out my hurt and my pain, hoping for some comfort and guidance. I had missed that so much since Josie's death. Something inside of me told me that I needed to get out. I think that was Josie's quiet whisper encouraging me to move on. I suppose that my prayers were answered because in her own special way, she was still guiding me. So Chris and I and the children who were now five and three and a half years old, went in search of our new home. Our 1930's two story, three bedroom house sold in thirty days and we had a bidding war to boot. So we needed to act quickly. It was a fun adventure and we found the perfect place to call our home. It is no coincidence that when something feels right, it just happens so easily. I remember walking into what would be our new home and thinking of mom right away. One look at the wainscoting in the hallway and the plaster swirls on the dining room ceiling, I thought, "Ma would love this house". My second thought was of Josie and how she would have loved a house like this one. It felt so right and the energy was uplifting, even though the couple who lived there was going their separate ways. I suppose everyone had a chance at a new beginning.

Chapter 46

The Other Sister

SISTERS. WHAT a blessing it is to have one. How unfortunate for those who don't. There are so many that long to have a sister to call their own. In my opinion this relationship takes second to the complexity of the mother-daughter relationship. It can be a genuinely rewarding experience or the biggest pain in the ass, and sometimes, all at the same time.

I have made many references to my sister Tina throughout, however my relationship with her is deserving of a chapter on its own. I feel that if I left out the less flattering parts, then I would not be doing justice to one of the most important relationships in my life.

We all know the concept of three is always a difficult one. "Three is a crowd" we would often hear when we were young. Someone was always the third one out and in our case that third one was me. I never felt the need to compete with my sister's relationship with one another. The age differences between us decided that for us. They were together and I somewhere off on my own. I had a very different relationship with each of them and I suppose that was based on our personalities and compatibilities. I am not sure. Maybe it's our genetics. Who knows?

The stories about Tina and her growing up bring a smile to all of our faces especially to the brothers who are older and remember her antics well. As many immigrant families do, dad came over first, set up shop and sent for mom who came to Canada in 1952 with the three boys. They all traveled by boat in those days. Imagine how long that took. Unfortunately, mom had a miscarriage with the twins. But then in 1954 she gave birth to a baby girl; a daughter her first of three. From the stories I have been told, mom was elated. Having a daughter after all these boys was a dream come true. But Tina was a little more than mom anticipated. She was a rather active child with a little mind of her own. She didn't sleep well and would often get up in the middle of the night with her pillow under her arm and lay herself down on the floor in the hallway. I am told that mom was either pregnant with Josie or just overall exhausted, but she would pick her up and bring her back to bed. Tina was co-operative and went back to her bed, only to return moments later when all was quiet and she thought mom was sound asleep. This would often continue throughout the night. I can only imagine how cute she was with that big pillow under her arm, her golden blonde hair and those pretty blue eyes.

My other favorite story is the one with the milk bottles. I remember my mother and father shaking their heads and telling us this story with a smile on their face. It was the fifties and there was a move away from breast feeding and into using bottles; especially plastic and many were using them. It seemed that this was the preferred bottle of choice for baby Tina too. She quickly discovered that if she squeezed the bottle then the milk would create fancy designs on the ceiling and on the walls. She had a real hoot and mom knew then that she had a very spirited child on her hands.

She was the oldest of the girls and the most gregarious. She and Josie were four days short of being a year apart. So they celebrated their birthdays together, shared a bedroom and even dressed alike. The blue blouse was usually given to Tina to match her blue eyes and Josie the green one because her eyes were hazel. Josie had a mild temperament and often preferred to be in the background. But Tina always needed to be in the center of it all. I often settle in and watch the old family movies and there she is, my sister Tina, organizing all the other kids for the photo shoots. Everyone needed to stand or sit where she had placed them and honestly it was always the right spot. She would have such a proud look on her face and a big smile knowing that she had contributed. Tina demonstrated excellent verbal and organizational skills at an early age. Right then and there, we knew that a teacher was born. Mom would be thrilled.

Tina has been a contributor for most of her life. She is definitely a giver and a doer. Being the oldest of the girls, Tina took on certain tasks that were assigned to her. She would learn to boil bottles, glass ones as it was now the sixties. She would feed me and help with my care. Mom also asked her to help with other chores as well as the cooking. In many ways, it all paid off because my sister keeps an immaculately clean house and as you already know, is an excellent cook.

Caring for me would prove to create friction and tension between me and Tina. I had often interpreted my sister's delegation of duties as bossiness and I wasn't in for that as I too had my own ideas of how things should be. Tina is a very loving and giving person but as a doer, she wants to do things herself and in her own way. Essentially she is no different than millions of us women out there. It's just that I was eight years younger and I didn't want anyone telling me what to do. Josie was always our buffer but she was not here anymore to smooth things over and soften the edges of her two stubborn sisters.

Despite our differences, nothing would prepare Tina and I for what life would be like after Josie's death. I know that in the months and even years, after Josie passed, our relationship was often conflicted. For the first time in my life, I felt that we were competing. Whose pain was deeper? Who felt the loss of Josie more? Was it Tina who shared a childhood of memories, or was it me, who had shared so many wonderful times as adults? Josie and I spoke three times a day and we laughed and did so many fun things together during those last years. I realize now and I feel that Tina does too, that we both had the privilege of having a sister who brought so much into our lives. What is it that we had to prove and to whom? All we have is our own memories of her and most importantly her children. We know that she loved her kids from the bottom of her heart and although her time with them was short, she gave them so much. It is through her children that we are still able to experience her love and so it becomes important that both Tina and I be near the children. What I have failed to understand is that for Tina, showing her love for them is doing for them and for me, showing my love is being with them. Neither of us is wrong and I hope that Josie's children have benefited from what we both have to give.

After all of these years without Josie in our lives, Tina and I have finally found our place with one another. We speak very little of the friction in our past but we both know it existed. We have a quiet understanding that our deep pain and sorrow over the loss of our sister turned on that ugly side of ourselves and at times made us turn our backs on each other. I am at peace that we have grown from that place. As we have mourned her loss, we have both come to understand and appreciate our own unique love for her. I know Josie would be happy and proud that we have joined together to do and to be there for her children.

Chapter 47

Saying Good Bye to Pa

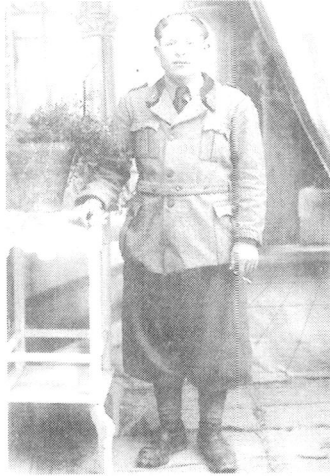

Pa in the Italian Army ~ 1939

WHEN THERE are six siblings in one family, it is often hard to maintain regular contact with each of them all the time. Different work schedules, kids and whatever else was going on made it difficult for us to call each other often. But we rarely worried about it because we knew that dad was keeping us all informed of what was going on in each other's lives.

Dad called this "keeping us all in communication". Yet we rarely missed our daily check in with him who we called Pa. We knew that he expected to hear from all of us daily. Even as adults he kept a tight rein on us all.

Despite all the heartache in dad's life, he lived into his eighty-eighth year. He died on January 9th 2001. It was my Nicole's fourth birthday. He spent his last eighteen months living with my sister Tina and her family. I knew that dad would always end up with Tina. Josie and I always called her the golden girl as Tina could do no wrong in dad's eyes. But all joking aside, he always felt a closeness to her and felt that she most resembled his own mother. I think that Tina gave dad that nurturing that he had lost so young in his life. It is her mothering nature that gave dad that comfort that he longed to have in his last years. I am grateful to Tina and her husband, Rocco and their children, Michael and Matthew, for opening their doors and providing dad with a loving place to rest.

About one year before dad died, I had taken him to a doctor's appointment and when I brought him back home to Tina's house, we sat and had a cup of tea together. He told me that he wanted to talk with me and with dad; you didn't always know what you were in for. My dad was a wonderful story teller but his downfall was that he took too long to tell the story. He would always take these long pauses and I have noticed that I have been doing the same lately. Anyways...... dad proceeded to tell me that there was a time when he felt that I had chosen the wrong path in my life. I was suddenly holding my breath, worried that he was about to throw the past in my face; again. He went on to explain that he did not know how to handle my strong personality and that he was struggling to be both mother and father to me. I am now thinking, where is he going with this? He wanted me to know that he realized that he was wrong. What! He proceeded to tell me that he has watched me with my children and is very proud of the woman and the mother that I have become. I was frozen. He then said that I was "La Regina di tutti li mamas". What! I am the queen of all mothers? I did not know what to say so I used my humor as a disguise to hide my true feelings. I do that often and I thanked dad for all the compliments. He told me that these were not meant to be compliments, but rather his feelings that came from his heart. I will never forget the way Pa and I looked at one another that day. I could feel his sincerity. I thanked Pa and told him how important it was for me to hear those words from him. I think that he knew that. I had waited my whole life to receive validation from my father. And that day was the day that I knew that if I never saw my father again, that we had made our peace. As it turned out, one year later they discovered that dad had stomach cancer too, only it was not the same type as Josie's cancer. It was a tumor and within the week, dad was gone.

We had just celebrated a beautiful Christmas which Chris and I hosted, when days later dad was rushed to the emergency. He had been losing blood but it seemed so gradual, none of us noticed that he had become so pale. After several tests to determine from where he was losing this blood, we learned that dad had a tumor in his stomach. We were shocked and had no idea. Apparently, neither did dad. I remember asking our much loved family doctor, Dr. R who has seen our family through our darkest times, how long Dad had this tumor? I found his response to be rather interesting. He stated that judging by the size; it looked like it had been there for about five years. I thought to myself that this was no coincidence given that Josie died six years ago. Naturally there is no way to prove my theory, at least not scientifically, but I believe that the excruciating pain dad felt over losing a daughter, so young and beautiful; a daughter who had no choice but to leave her three gentle angels behind, led to his illness. Where does all that raw emotion go? In my opinion, it can turn all that suffering into disease and in dad's case, it led to his death.

I remember the days in the hospital leading up to dad's final days. He was slipping in and out and I was wondering where he was and who he was with. By this point, I had done some research on the spirit world and had a few experiences with the other side of my own. As he lay on the hospital bed, I heard dad talking and he sounded so happy as if he had seen someone that he had not seen in a long time. I heard him calling out the names of his loved ones. I was sure that they had come for him to take him to this glorious place called Heaven. I heard him say,

"Rosa Bella, it's been so long since I have seen you". Even though dad had a sister named Rosa that had died years ago, I knew that standing before him was his own beautiful rose. He was talking to Josie. I knew that she had come for Pa. I sat so still and so close to him in hopes that I could somehow catch a glimpse of her too. I was afraid to move because I did not want to break the moment. All of a sudden dad opened his eyes and I asked him, who did you see? Was it Josie? Dad smiled and lovingly said to me "You always want to know things that you should not know". I suppose that is one of my characteristics that drove dad crazy for all of these years. But I knew by his look that they were all there with Josie to help dad pass over. His mother and father who had abandoned him by dying an early death, his sister and of course his wife, our mother, who had died and left dad twenty years ago.

Dad`s death was one of the least tragic that I have ever experienced. He had lived a long life full of happiness and sorrow and he died with all of his children around his bed. The outlaws were there too. Dad considered them to be like his own children and they too looked to Pa as their own father. He even said his goodbyes to his grandchildren whom he loved so much and reminded them to keep on the right path. I was right beside dad as he lay on his death bed and could hear his every breath. After all that Pa and I had been through, I too had earned my spot to be there with him until the end. Despite what dad and my siblings may have thought of my decisions in my early twenties, I was a good daughter and a loving daughter and I had every right to be by his side.

Chapter 48

Last Call to Sammy

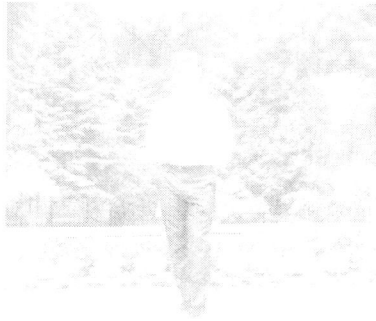

My brother Sammy

WE NO longer have dad to" keep everyone in communication", so we have to do it ourselves. Honestly, I think that dad would be proud as Sunday mornings are designated for talking on the phone. The first call is usually from my brother Joe. He is the oldest and since dad's passing, he is considered the patriarch of the family. Finally after several years, my sister Tina and I have trained him to call after ten am. Every now and then he calls a little earlier and asks, "Did I get you out of bed". He knows that really pisses me off.

Years of getting up at the crack of dawn with kids and then up for work early everyday of the week, I feel that I am entitled to stay in bed for as long as the good Lord will let me sleep. Of course now, I can't sleep in even if I wanted to. So when he says that to me, I smile and say "Of course not. I have been up for hours". Then we laugh. He is the oldest, and I the youngest with twenty two years between us. He and Doris have raised three sons and have grandchildren too. We talk about many things and I have learned so much about him in the last years. I have also learned that of all of my siblings, I think that I am the most like him. We share a common drive for adventure and an enthusiasm for life. Neither of us is afraid to take a risk.

As for Tina and I, we carve out some time to talk on Sunday mornings or anytime of the week for that matter. We discuss the comings and goings of what is happening in our lives and within the family and yes, we both like to analyze.

My brother John and I have always maintained a close connection with one another. John is a very sweet and soft spoken man but has a very stubborn streak. He has been retired for several years now as work was becoming more difficult with his arthritic knees. We are still trying to convince him to have a knee replacement but he is so stubborn. He lives with pain everyday and I hate the thought of him suffering so much. I love my brother Johnny. He and his wife Cynthia have two beautiful children, Jessica and Andrew who are kind and respectful individuals. I am so grateful that I have come to really know them and love them.

As for my brother Sammy, he was never much for talking on the telephone His conversations were often brief. But he had some of the best one liners that often said it all. He used words like "peachy" and called me "squirt" My brother Sammy was a kind man and although he seemed rough around the edges, he had a huge heart and like Josie, had a

227

very playful side to him. After mom died, an aneurism struck when Sam was in his early forties and he was never the same. Sam was a laborer for most of his life and never shied away from hard work. After several surgeries and assessments, it was determined that Sam would never work again. This was devastating news for a man who always worked hard to provide for his wife, Angela and their three daughters. But Sam tried to make the best of those years despite feeling angry and bitter that life had dealt him such a bitter hand. For years he tried to drown his feelings deeper and deeper. Sam was never one to talk much about his feelings. "That is sissy stuff," he would say. But we all knew how sensitive he was particularly when mom died. After her death, he stated that he did not want to ever talk about mom again or even speak her name. I think the pain of losing mom lasted a lifetime for Sam. I don't think he ever recovered from her loss.

When Josie died, he couldn't speak. None of us could. Then, he surprised us all and after years and years of smoking very strong cigarettes, he quit. We were all so happy. Dad would have been very proud of him. He was even coming around more at many of the family gatherings. I remember feeling that maybe Sam had a new lease on life. But soon after, he was diagnosed with lung cancer and on June 8th 2009, he died at the age of sixty-five. Somehow I am thinking that Sam's diagnosis came long before he was even prepared to tell anyone. Despite his lengthy illness, Sam died suddenly. It just occurred to me how a man like my brother, who kept his painful feelings inside, his whole life, died because he choked on the blood of a lung that exploded inside of him. I suppose that I don't even need to ask the question of where all of Sam's raw emotions went. It is fairly clear to me.

To this day, I am so grateful that I listened to that little voice inside my head telling me to call my brother. I had phoned Sammy four hours before he collapsed and died. I asked him how he was doing? He answered "Just peachy". Who knew that this would be the last call I would ever make to my brother Sammy. When I think of him now, I remember his handsome face, blonde curls and his true blue eyes. I see a lot of him in my own son, Mitchell.

My fondest memories of my brother Sam are when he took me shoe shopping. It does seem rather odd that a rugged guy like Sam would do such a thing. But I had decided that I wanted a pair of Dr. Scholl's exercise sandals; the wooden ones with a brown strap. We went all over the downtown core to find a pair of these in a size one. Sam's determination paid off because we found them. I was thrilled and so was he. On one of our other shopping excursions, he took me everywhere to find a white pair of Go Go boots. Of course it was the sixties and they were the latest in fashion. This time, Sam decided that I had to have a pair and we found the perfect ones. What is it about my brother Sam and shoes? I am reminded by Tina that when she and Josie were little girls, Sam would pay them "two bits" which was his way of saying a quarter, if they shinned his black leather pointed toe shoes. Oh, Sammy was always so full of life and energy. When memories are all you have, you thank God that you have some really special ones.

Chapter 49

The Red Cardinal

July 4th 2012 I write

Good Morning My Dearest Josie,

I decided to write to you this morning. After all, you are my angel. It has been so long since I have taken the time to write and there is so much that I want to say. A lot has been going on and I know that I need to settle myself and find some time for peace and quiet. It is actually quite early in the morning. I know that you are killing yourself laughing because you remember the days when I used to be up all night and sleep late into the morning, while you were up early with your three little angels. As they say, "What goes around comes around." I too had my turn at being up with my two little darlings, particularly with the one who loved to get up at the crack of dawn. Now that they are older, I can sleep in until noon if I wanted to, but I can't. I suppose it's part of getting older.

I actually enjoy being the first one up. Imagine!
It is true what all those morning early birds say.
There is something peaceful about the morning.
I think it is the freshness of the air and the calm-
ness of our surroundings that help us to heal
our spirit. Everything is so still and all you can
hear is the chirping sounds of the birds. They
are so beautiful and we have noticed so many
of them in our backyard. I had mentioned this
to a lovely spiritual lady friend and she told me
that the birds keep coming because they are
attracted to our energy. Chris and I decided to
dig out the bird feeder that the kids and I bought
for him ages ago for Father's Day. Chris keeps
filling it with bird seed and naturally, they just
keep coming. What a blessing to see so many
lovely birds visiting every day. We are talking a
lot of beautiful birds, like the ones in your school
project. I have a confession to make. I am sure
that you already know but, I copied that bird
project years later and traced all of your beautiful pictures. I got a really good mark on that too.
I am sure that you have already forgiven me.
Anyways, every time one of these birds comes
around, I think of you. I know it's crazy!

One day this beautiful red Cardinal came
around and stayed for quite awhile, like about
two weeks. I know that the Cardinal was your
favorite bird but, there was something special
about this one. Chris suspected that there was
a nest nearby and I think he was right. This
Cardinal was rather brave and came right up
to our deck and perched itself on the back of

the patio chair. You know, the wicker rocking chairs that I have always longed to sit in with you sipping tea and talking like we used to at your house. We never got a chance to do that at my house even though I have pictured us so vividly in my mind. I started to tell the family about these regular visits and naturally we were all intrigued because we all know that birds bring messages and good news. I think Ma told us that long ago. There has been much speculation since this bird's arrival. Tina and I have analyzed it every which way possible. But it all really remains a mystery and anyways we had a shower to plan.

The bridal shower for Anthony's bride Mary Anne was fast approaching and the "committee", you know who you are, was very busy with the final arrangements and set up. The shower was to be at my house and it was a lovely event. The weather could have been better but let's focus on the positives and there were many. It was a lovely coming together of both families and Mary Anne was beautiful and beaming. Our tea party theme was a success. We gave everyone the tea cup that they used at the shower to take home. We had a beautiful selection of cups. I know that you would have loved it. Andrea was right in there every step of the way. She is a beauty. She is a lot like you but she also has her own special something. I know that you are with her all the time because I see it and I feel it when I am around her. There were several sightings of the Cardinal on the day of the shower. Anthony even mentioned seeing the Cardinal.

The next day I was spent and decided to take the day off since I couldn't walk and hadn't taken a day off work in ages. So I stayed home and relaxed in the backyard. Of course the weather was great on the Monday, but in keeping with my positive thoughts, I decided to take what I could of the day and reflect on what a successful shower we were able to give to Anthony and his bride. I looked around and noticed that the Cardinal was nowhere to be found. There were many birds as per usual going back and forth to the bird feeder, but no red Cardinal. It was the strangest thing, but I felt such a sense of loss. I had not said anything to anyone for fear of sounding like a silly woman. But I casually asked Chris if he had seen the Cardinal and much to my surprise, he too had not seen the Cardinal and he sounded disappointed. Anyway, life goes on and after a couple of days, I decided I was well enough to go back to work.

Two weeks had passed and still no red bird! I know it sounds unbelievable, but when this Cardinal took shelter in our backyard, it could be seen and heard from everywhere in our house. If I was upstairs in my bedroom, I would hear its distinct chirp so I would look out the window and there it was. If I was in my favorite room in the house, the sitting room, I would hear it, look out the bay window and there it was, perched on the neighbor's roof looking at me through the window. Even Quinney and our old mama cat, Wheetzie, love this Cardinal because they never made any attempt to capture it. They obviously knew that there was something special about this bird. We all did, but we just didn't know what it was for sure. I frequently sit in the backyard listening to the sounds of summer and watch the beautiful birds coming and going. I do miss our beautiful red Cardinal and keep hoping that someday soon; it will stop by for a visit.

Chapter 50

What I Know Now at 50

I TURNED FIFTY this year and was showered with gifts and celebrations that really meant a lot to me. There was definitely a show of love from my family and very close friends. What a blessing to have reached this milestone. I have never feared getting older. It's more that I never really imagined myself at this age. If it wasn't for the aches and pains and the fact that I can no longer see what is right in front of me, I would think that I am twenty-five. There are times when I think back to what my life was like at that age. Songs on the retro station and fashion that has come back in style, bring back such vivid memories of the days when we left the house after nine to stand outside in the lineup, in the winter with no coat, to get into the hottest dance club in the city. We would dance and dance all night. Those were great times. We worried about finding Mr. Right and what our future had in store for us.

I remember Josie always telling me that I worried too much and that I was a deep thinker, too deep for her. Josie never liked to analyze things too much. She felt I over analyzed everything and I suppose she was right. I guess it was my process in trying to understand the things that were going on around me. Now as I get older, I feel that I am more reflective and I think to myself, ``Who really knows what life has in store for us?'' I would have never guessed at that time, that life with Josie as we knew it, would come to an end in less than ten years. Josie's illness and her subsequent death affected so many people because others identified with her and her life. She was a soccer mom and took on an active role on parent council at the school where her children attended. She was always doing for others. She maintained a positive attitude and rarely saw the negative in anyone. People were thinking, if this could happen to Josie, it could happen to me. That is often the reality when people in the prime of their lives with young families die.

I have learned through my life experiences and all the losses that I have endured, especially Josie's, that life is precious and that every year is really a bonus. I have also learned so much from Josie's life. I have had the privilege of knowing her and loving her. Despite the pain and sadness from all of those years, I know that I am a better person for having her in my life. She taught me to see the light in others. I know that my relationship with her children is richer and that her memory lives through them. Josie's life had purpose. She taught me and others how to love and how to receive and embrace love. She showed so much strength.

There is such power within a family and a tragedy such as this one, can either strengthen the bond or weaken it. We have all come out stronger. I understand the things in life that really matter and have surrounded myself with people that love and support me. I am human and there are moments that I still feel bitter about the loss of my family members. During those moments I cherish my beautiful memories of them and remind myself of the privilege I had in being a part of this family. I have been fortunate in my life that I have always known the power and the value of communication. In the early days, I gave my mother the opportunity to express herself and her feelings toward her terminal cancer. At that time, and for that matter, during the time of Josie's illness, there were no support groups. Fortunately, organizations have now realized that group support helps people who are affected by cancer know that they are not alone. I have always felt this ache that I could not give that support to Josie. For so many years I have been feeling like I was not there for her to really listen to her fears. I was so stuck in my own fear of losing her that I felt like I let her down.

In going through this process of writing My Journey with Josie, I finally realize that I did not let her down. I was there for her in the ways that she needed. We did talk about her fears, but we just didn't over analyze them! It's not who she was. For Josie, it was more important for her to live out her life in the way that mattered to her the most and that was to be a loving mother, a devoted wife, a trusting sister, a caring daughter and a loyal friend. Talking about her fears was not what she needed from me.

I recently met with two of Josie's dearest friends Marnie and Franca. We laughed and cried as we thought about the times when Josie was in our lives. What I learned the most about my time with them was not what I had expected. I suppose it was what I was meant to, and I have no doubt, that it was what Josie had intended for me to know. I learned that I made a difference in Josie's life. She cared for me and what was going on in my life and all the drama in it. I always felt that I was taking from her and not giving her anything in return. Did I in some way contribute to her stress by dumping all my conflicts with dad on her? I learned that Josie felt it was her role as my older sister to advocate and protect my honor after I left the family home. She loved me as much as I loved her. I ask myself what have I learned from Josie's passing, or moms, dads and Sammy's for that matter?

How has it changed me? I have learned that cancer is not something that you deserve, it just happens. It is not a punishment for being a bad person. Just as grieving is not God's way to punish us through suffering. What could I have possibly done in my life that would justify the magnitude of my pain? What wrong did Josie's children do to deserve a life without their loving mother? Absolutely nothing. We can continue to debate the reasons why but after all the losses in my life I still do not know why. To me that answer will remain a mystery. That is not to say that I have not gone in search for the answer. But I have come away with a knowing that there is something greater, a higher spiritual being that sends messages of love and gives us a sign that there is life beyond our current world. I am so grateful that I have been touched by spirit and have experienced the comfort that it brings. I have been able to share my love and experiences with Josie's children and together with the family, we have done our best to keep Josie's memory alive in them just as she had requested of us so many years ago.

Anthony, Paul and Andrea have grown up and have never forgotten the greatness that their mother instilled in them. They are responsible, caring and loving individuals that Josie would be proud of. Each has traveled down their own path which at times has not been easy. The boys have gone on to form their families and creating children of their own to complete the family life cycle. Andrea continues her journey as a motherless daughter and is embracing the many possibilities that the future holds for her. Together, as Josie's sisters, Tina and I continue to give her and the boys our love and our guidance.

I know that even at fifty, I will always be the baby of this generation of offspring. I have embraced this role and along with my husband and children have opened up our hearts and our home and brought the family together to enjoy and celebrate life and all it has to offer. Together as a family, we have experienced the loss of our parents and siblings and know how important it is to treasure each other. Being the youngest of the family, I know that there will be a time when I will have to say good bye to my remaining siblings and that will not be easy. I have been fortunate enough to come from a place where we have learned the value of family and I will be forever grateful to my parents for giving that to us.

Despite my unexpected hysterectomy and ongoing meno-pausal ordeal, I am grateful that I have been given good health and strong stamina in my life. At fifty, I know that I have yet a lot more to accomplish. I am on a journey to free myself of all that has held me back in my life. I am learning that I have the power within myself to do great things and I am slowly chipping away at my fears. I am grateful for my husband and children and I am blessed with having so many of my nieces and nephews who show me their love and seek my guidance. They along with my own children are the new generation of this family.

I have learned that I am the greatest gift to myself and I am taking the time to nurture and feed my soul. I have offi-cially become an early morning bird and continue to enjoy the peaceful surroundings of my backyard. I recently found myself looking and listening for my red Cardinal. I was think-ing about when I last saw the Cardinal and how close it made me feel to Josie. I wondered if I would ever see this Cardinal again and whether it would connect me spiritually to her. As absurd as this may sound, I asked Josie to show herself to me by giving me a sign. I thought to myself that if the Cardinal returned, then this would be my proof that Josie is near. A part of me was feeling like I was really losing touch with reality, but the larger part of me didn't care and I was hoping that this beautiful red bird would reappear.

It was a gorgeous day and I felt the warmth of the sun all around me but I was protected by the canopy and enjoyed the summer breeze. I had not felt this relaxed in a long while. I closed my eyes and let my head rest on the back of the wicker rocking chair. It was so quiet and peaceful and I felt like I could doze off at any moment when suddenly, I felt compelled to open my eyes. I could not believe what I was seeing. Perched on the bird feeder was this beautiful red Cardinal, my Cardinal. Not showing any interest in the seed, the Cardinal just stared at me and I stared back. I tried to catch my breath but I did not want to move because I wanted to stay in this moment with her forever. My heart was beating so fast and before I knew it, the Cardinal turned around and shook its tale as if it were waving at me. I knew that this was Josie's sense of humor. I always loved that playful side to her and obviously that cheekiness we so loved, is still with her in spirit. I was laughing out loud and that brought me out of the moment. I laughed some more and then she darted off into the sky. I have not seen my red Cardinal since, but I know that I am never alone for she is always near and never far.

Letters To Mom

IN WRITING My Journey with Josie, I wanted to give her children the opportunity to express their love for their mother and their feelings about living life without her. We agreed that writing a letter to their mother would be a meaningful way to communicate their deepest thoughts and feelings. In the following pages, I have included Anthony and Andrea letters to their mother. They have embraced the opportunity to share these feelings with my readers. Paul however at this time has chosen to keep his personal thoughts and feelings private. I wish all three of Josie's children a life of peace, joy and happiness knowing that their mother is always near.

Dear Mom,

> I didn't realize how hard it would be to put my thoughts and feelings on paper. When Aunt Sal asked me to write something for her book I was honored and I thought this was going to be easy. However, when I sat down to actually do it I found myself staring at the keyboard with nothing to say. Now I know how you felt when aunt Sal handed you that journal knowing that we would read it someday. I'll try to be a little more descriptive than you were though.

It's been 18 years since I've heard your voice and to this day I swear I hear you calling my name when no one is around. You've missed a lot since you've been gone. The first few years were the hardest. Everyone tried so hard to keep us busy and entertained like nothing had changed, but everything had changed. My world crumbled all around me, and not even a friendly mouse or a magical castle could change that. Not to say that I didn't appreciate what everyone did, but I would have traded it all for one more day with you.

Dad put up a good front but he was never the same. A part of him was gone and now he was responsible for raising 3 kids on his own. It took a toll on him because I think loosing you was almost too much for him to bear. Thank God for Elsa though, she was fantastic. Elsa was there for us every day after school. She made a mean bowl of soup and she didn't hesitate to let us know when we were getting out of line. I owe her so much. She taught me how to take care of myself. Before her, I didn't even know what the inside of the washing machine looked like. She was a very wise woman who obviously knew that she wouldn't be there to take care of us forever and that at some point, we would have to fend for ourselves. She was right.

Eventually Dad met someone and it progressed pretty quickly. But life was never the same. For the next 10 years, I felt like no one cared where I was or what I was doing; and I took full advantage of that. My life had changed, and at the time, I didn't realize just how much. I tried to stay positive and I tried to hold on to the values that you instilled in me, but day by day, and year by year, I got covered in this hard exterior. It's hard to stay positive when you are constantly exposed to negativity. It was also difficult to feel happiness when I realized just how much I had lost in my life. I had an opportunity to move out on my own and I jumped at it, even though I was far from ready.

I was 26 years old but I still felt like that 13 year old boy who desperately missed his mom. I was empty inside and it seemed like nothing could make me whole again. I was on my own, staying out till all hours of the night, drinking, gambling and a whole list of thing that don't need mentioning. No matter what I did or how dark things got, I always knew you were there looking out for me because if you weren't, I know I wouldn't be here today. I may not have made the best choices in my life but each of them helped me become the man I am today.

Now I'm 31 years old and I've separated myself from all of the negative influences in my life. It wasn't easy and some feelings were hurt along the way, but I'm better for it and I feel like a huge weight has been lifted off my shoulders. I'm in a better place.

I'm married to the most wonderful woman in the world. Mary-Anne has shown me that it's ok to share my feelings and now I can actually

talk about you without feeling the uncontrol-
lable urge to cry. She has a way of lighting a
fire under me. She is my life's purpose. She has
helped me find my voice and she brings out the
best in me.

Mary-Anne has the most beautiful little daughter named Ava. Her face lights up a room and
there's nothing I wouldn't do for her. I may not
have had a hand in making her, but regardless, she's my daughter until the day I die. As
I'm sure you know we just had a little boy. We
named him Luca Joseph. As I'm writing this, he
is 2 weeks old and the most precious little thing.
I show him your picture all the time. It makes
me sad to think that he'll never get the chance
to meet his Nonna. My only hope is that I can
show Luca and Ava the same love and devotion
that you showed me when I was growing up.

If I've learned anything over the last 18 years
it's that moving on is different than forgetting.
You can't sit around feeling sorry for yourself
because time will keep on ticking, and the world
will keep on spinning. If you are not careful,
before you know it your life will have passed you
by. For me it only took just one person to open
my eyes and show me that life was still worth
living. She has given me a family of my own and
all the love and support that I had been missing
for so long. For that, I am eternally grateful.

I've spent more than half of my life without you
now. Not a day goes by that I haven't thought
about you or wondered what my life would have

been like if you were still with me. I've come to realize that everything I've been through has brought me here. If I hadn't had those experiences, I wouldn't be the man I am today. I wouldn't trade my family for anything. I try to live each day with the knowledge and faith that you are still by my side and I try to express that in everything I do. It is the only way I know how to keep your memory and values alive in my children, and most importantly, myself. So you can rest easy mom, it may have taken a while, but now I know I'm going to be ok. I love you...

Anthony

Dear Mom,

This is going to be one major therapy session for me. I haven't even started yet and I have a tear running down my cheek. As I sit here on my bed, I look on my nightstand—two books that I have been wanting to crack open but I have always made excuses. Both books are about mothers who are not in their children's lives... come to think of it; maybe my excuses are really my fears. I've decided that my contribution to my aunt's book will be a letter to my mother; a compilation of all the things that I want to tell her.

Mom,

You know how people say "this is the hardest letter I've ever had to write" Either they are lying or they have never written a letter to their dead mother. Beginning this letter with the word mom is so very strange to me. I rarely write the word, I never say it, and when I do, it's like I am speaking a different language. I haven't been able to call for you for eighteen years, I mean, I can call for you all I want but I am never going to get an answer. I don't even know if that's what I would call you if you were still alive. Would I call you 'Mom'? 'Ma'? 'Mommy'? Would we have funny little names picked out for each other? Who knows, I'll just call you mom for simplicities sake.

My memories of you only date back so far. I was six when you died so these memories are becoming more and more blurred to me and I am afraid I will forget them as time goes on so maybe it's good that I have this chance to write everything down. I will warn you, there are exactly five memories that I have of you where I can remember exactly where I was and what I was doing. I only wish I could remember your face or hear your voice because every time I try to imagine it, nothing happens. The first memory I have of you is when we used to spend our days together while dad was at work and Anthony and Paul were at school. We had the days to ourselves. I was little so we probably played with my toys or something but now that I am older, I often wonder what we would spend our time doing. Probably shopping, baking (an interest I *know* I got from you), pampering, and I'm sure some mother daughter arguing would take place. But on this particular day we had a bath. You filled up the tub, not too much (I was and still am afraid of water...something else I *know* I got from you!) and you always put in an insane amount of bubbles. These bubbles were an essential part of this bath experience because we used to make dresses out of them. There I was, at the drain end of the tub and you on the other and we would cover ourselves in bubbles and see who could make the prettiest dress. I'm sure I always won. This may seem like a silly memory to hold on to, but it is something I think I'd do with my daughter...if I have one.

My second memory is closely related to the bubble bath beauty boutique, it could have easily followed or it could have been a completely different day. I am not sure. You were at the kitchen table on the phone (probably with one of your sisters) and you had a towel wrapped around you. It wasn't wrapped around your shoulders, but it was wrapped around under your arms. So, I wanted to do the same. I stood right in front of you and tried to mirror your towel wrapping technique. The key word in that sentence is *tried* because right after I *tried* it, you told me that I needed boobs to do that. Ya! You heard me! I was so upset from that day on, I always wished for big boobs and I guess now that I have them I shouldn't have wished that hard.

My third memory is one that you do not know about...but I guess now you do. I was sick one day and needed to take medicine and you remember how much of a hassle it was to get me to take my medicine. Well, it was taking me so long to take this little cupful of liquid. You told me that if I wasn't finished it by the time you got back from the bathroom, I would be in big trouble. So, while you went and did your business, I, like any other intelligent 5 year old dumped the medicine down the kitchen sink! You were very pleased with me when you returned thinking that I took the medicine and I thought I was the sneakiest child in the world. I never did end up telling you the truth and apologizing for what I did that day so I will say it now. I'm sorry.

My fourth memory is one tiny snapshot. In our kitchen there was a blue wooden stool in the corner underneath the telephone. I just remember always dragging this stool to the counter where you were either cooking or baking and wanting to help you or just see what you were doing.

My last memory of you was when you were in the hospital. I am not sure how sick you were but I remember you telling me to crawl into the hospital bed with you. I was so scared. I was afraid that I was going to hurt you or break one of the tubes that you were hooked up to. I did end up coming onto the bed but I was not at all comfortable...I'm sure you weren't either.

When you were diagnosed with the monster of all monsters, I was four years old. I don't even know if I was told that you had cancer, and if I was, I know I didn't know what it all meant.

I remember you coming home from the hospital and I thought, "Ok good. She's home for good now" I have never been more wrong in my life. May 14th 1995 is now the day I wish never existed. I hate that day even more when Mother's Day falls on it. Mother's Day fell on it that year. How convenient. I left for school that day with not a care in the world and came home to something that would shape every part of my being for the rest of my life. I was so excited to come home that afternoon to give you all the things I made for you at school for Mother's Day but when I opened the door, you weren't on the couch where I had last seen you. After that, it's all a blur. I don't know if that's the last time I saw you alive. It probably was because the next memory I have is someone (I don't know who) telling me, "She almost beat the pain, but the pain beat her." I don't know where I was when I was told that but I know the image that went through my head and its one that I can still see to this day. I pictured a stadium filled with people and they were cheering, they were all cheering for you, Mom. You were in a race with a giant blob of green goop. May I just add that this entire vision was in cartoon...that just goes to show how young I actually was and how I interpreted all of this. Anyway, you looked so tired and so drained and this blob had slid its way passed the finish line a split second before you did. I wish you came in first place.

I don't remember anything about the ceremony at the church although I would like to read your eulogy... I should look into that. I do remember wearing a red suit. Red bell bottom pants with a vest like shirt with round gold buttons down the front. I remember you wearing red that day too. I liked how we matched and I still have that outfit in a tote somewhere in this bedroom of mine. Your viewing is my first memory of you gone. When it was my turn to go up to your casket, I took my little left hand and touched your right. I was shocked to find that your hand was freezing; it didn't make sense to me. At the time I thought maybe you should be wearing a sweater. I'm not sure what made me want to reach out to touch you but the more I think about it, I'm glad I did.

The burial was the last thing I remember which makes sense because that was the last time I would ever be able to be near you. I walked up to your casket with Nonno. That's the exact time I learned that a parent should never bury their child. We held hands walking up to you and each put a flower on your casket. Now when I go to the cemetery I have flashbacks about walking up and down that path to and from your casket and it creeps me out a little. I don't go there much anymore and I'm sorry for that but as time goes on it seems to get harder and harder for me...something I didn't expect. I thought this was supposed to get easier.

When I was growing up I never really considered how much losing you would affect my life but as I get older I see why I am the way I am. I guess you could have called me a "tomboy" when I was growing up. I went from wearing dresses to school every day to wearing tear ways and tee shirts. I didn't wear a speck of makeup until I was 18 years old...mostly because I didn't know how to apply it. To this day I have a hard time shopping and putting outfits together and I always think that I'd have a knack for it if I had a mom. I could be wrong but I seem to dwell on things like these. Only recently have I started to take more of an active role in the way I look because I know that now is the time that I need to start acting and looking my age. I think I'm doing ok.

I used to try to reason with myself that losing you when I was so young was a good thing. I used to tell myself that because I was so young I didn't really have anything to miss about you because I didn't remember anything 'significant'. As I got older I quickly started to realize that I was very wrong. It's harder not knowing anything about you because I am left to think about the "what if's" and all the milestones in my life that you missed and will miss. I have a whole list in my head that haunts me and that makes me angry at the fact that you left me. You weren't there to pick out my communion dress with me. You missed my grade eight graduation and seeing me go through high school. You missed my two university graduations, my first serious boyfriend, you don't know who my best friends are and you're going to miss everything to come. My career and my wedding, my first house and my first child. I hate knowing that you won't be there for any of that and I hate knowing that we won't be able to make any memories together.

I also get scared about getting older because of you. With every year that passes I am closer to the age you were when you died. I get so scared that the same thing is going to happen to me. I am afraid that I will get sick and leave behind my husband and my kids like you did. The times I do think like this, which aren't that often, I usually give my head a shake and tell myself to stop thinking so negatively. Sometimes I just can't help it.

Besides all of the things that I know we won't get to share together, I know that in spirit, you will always be by my side. I am not mad at you any more for leaving me Mom. I've accepted it but I will forever have a scar on my heart. I know you would be proud of the woman I have become. I have a great life. I have an amazing family and the best friends anyone could ask for. I'm a teacher too Mom! I love my job and I love my life and not one day goes by that I don't think about what it would be like with you in it. One day, if I have a daughter of my own, I promise I will love her the way I know you loved me and I will do everything I can to be the mom you wanted to be for me.

Love you forever and ever, your little girl,

Andrea xoxo

Author's Note

MY SINCERE gratitude for taking the time and being a part of My Journey with Josie. As you know, writing this book has been a labor of love and a very personal journey for me. Use this page to write your comments, questions or whatever personal thoughts you may have. In the following pages, I have included discussion questions to enhance your group conversations about My Journey with Josie.

I invite you to visit my website at www.geturlifeon.ca if you wish to share your thoughts and experiences with me.

Thank you,

Salvina

Discussion Questions for Book Clubs and Support Groups

1. Do you feel that the author's worry about having cancer, prior to her hysterectomy, was an over-reaction or a valid concern given her family history?

2. The author describes how she was deeply impacted by the loss of her mother and years later by Josie's death. What are the parallels between these two losses?

3. Josie says in her journal, "Cancer was always the scariest word I knew. Now it was to become my whole life". In your opinion, how do you feel Josie coped with her terminal illness?

4. What are your thoughts about Josie's decision to stop her chemotherapy?

5. Do you feel that Josie's use of natural healing methods was beneficial? If so, in what way?

6. At what age are we ready to live without a mother? A father? A sibling?

7. Do you feel that as a mother, Josie could have done more for her children in her last ten months of her life?

8. Do you feel that there were any unresolved issues or

feelings between the author and Josie? What about between other family members and Josie?

9. In chapter 22, the author discusses the stages of dying. Do you feel that Josie and her family members went through these stages?

10. People go through many painful experiences in a lifetime. Where does all of that pain go?

11. Everyone grieves the loss of a loved one differently. Discuss the ways in which the author grieved the loss of Josie? How did other family members grieve?

12. Does one ever really accept the loss of a loved one?

13. What are your thoughts about the author's relationship with her other sister, Tina? How do you feel they were able to bridge the gap in their relationship without Josie?

14. Losing a child at any age is devastating. Do you feel that Josie's father could have developed his cancer as a result of his daughter's loss?

15. The author speaks of her family keeping their mother's diagnosis of cancer from her. Do you feel that she had a right to know?

16. From your perspective, how do you feel cancer has changed from the 70's to the 80's, the 90's to the 2000's?

17. In the section, Letters to Mom, two of Josie's children discuss their feelings about mother-loss. How do you feel they have been most impacted?

18. The author speaks honestly of her love and conflict with her father. Do you believe that they resolved their issues before he died?

19. Both the author and Josie talk about being touched by Spirit. What are your thoughts about their experiences?

20. Do you feel that the author's angel writings were help-

ful? If so, how?

21. What support systems were available to Josie throughout her fight for her life?

22. In the chapter, Last Call to Sammy, the author acted upon her intuition to call her brother not knowing that hours later he would die. Is this a coincidence or divine intervention? What are your thoughts and experiences?

23. In what ways has the author moved forward to live her life in a meaningful way without Josie?

About the Author

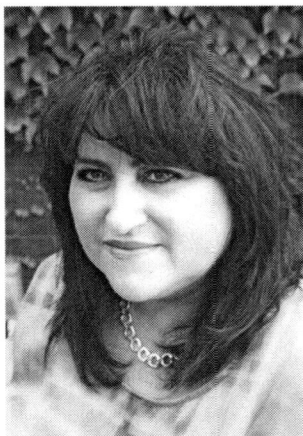

SALVINA GRICE is the youngest of six children -an Italian family whose parents emigrated from Racalmuto, Sicily, to Canada in the early 1950's. After graduating with Bachelor degrees in Social Work and Sociology from McMaster University in Hamilton, Ontario, Salvina has worked in various settings helping children and their families face life's challenges. She also has co founded an organization called Life Change with her husband Christopher, to further her practice in the private sector.

Salvina considers her most important role as being a mother to her two teenaged children, from which she draws inspiration to write about family life. Currently she is working on her second book titled Baby M.

For more information, visit her website at:
www.geturlifeon.ca.

CPSIA information can be obtained at www.ICGtesting.com
Printed in the USA
LVOW08s0621170414

381999LV00001B/19/P

9 781460 232484